DEVELOPING GROUNDED THEORY

The Second Generation

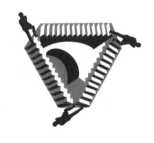

Developing Qualitative Inquiry

Series Editor: Janice M. Morse
University of Utah

Book in the new Developing Qualitative Inquiry series, written by leaders in qualitative inquiry, will address important topics in qualitative methods. Targeted to a broad multidisciplinary readership, the books are intended for mid-level/advanced researchers and advanced students. The series will forward the field of qualitative inquiry by describing new methods or developing particular aspects of established methods.

Volumes in this series:

1. Autoethnography as Method, Heewon Chang

2. Interpretive Description, Sally Thorne

3. Developing Grounded Theory: The Second Generation, Janice M. Morse, Phyllis Noerager Stern, Juliet Corbin, Barbara Bowers, Kathy Charmaz, Adele E. Clarke

DEVELOPING GROUNDED THEORY
THEORY
The Second Generation

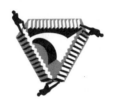

Janice M. Morse
Phyllis Noerager Stern
Juliet Corbin
Barbara Bowers
Kathy Charmaz
Adele E. Clarke

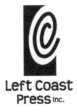

Left Coast
Press Inc.

Walnut Creek, California

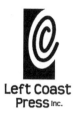

Left Coast Press Inc.

LEFT COAST PRESS, INC.
1630 North Main Street, #400
Walnut Creek, CA 94596
http://www.LCoastPress.com

Copyright © 2009 by Left Coast Press, Inc.

ISBN 978-1-59874-192-6 hardcover
ISBN 978-1-59874-193-3 paperback

Library of Congress Cataloging-in-Publication Data
Developing grounded theory : the second generation / Janice M. Morse ...[et al.].
    p. cm. -- (Developing qualitative inquiry)
  Includes index.
  ISBN 978-1-59874-192-6 (hardcover : alk. paper) – ISBN 978-1-59874-193-3 (pbk. : alk. paper)
  1. Grounded theory. I. Morse, Janice M.
  H61.24.D48 2008 2009
  001.4'2–dc22
                     2008048710

Printed in the United States of America

♾ ™ The paper used in this publication meets the minimum requirements of American National Standard for Information Sciences—Permanence of Paper for Printed Library Materials, ANSI/NISO Z39.48–1992.

09 10 11 12 5 4 3 2 1

CONTENTS

Preface: The Banff Symposium   9

Chapter 1: Tussles, Tensions, and Resolutions   13
    Janice M. Morse
    Dialogue: Doing "Grounded Theory"   21

Chapter 2: In the Beginning Glaser and Strauss   24
    Created Grounded Theory
    Phyllis Noerager Stern
    Photo Album   30

Chapter 3: Taking an Analytic Journey   35
    Juliet Corbin
    Dialogue: On "Cleaning" Transcripts   54

Chapter 4: Glaserian Grounded Theory   55
    Phyllis Noerager Stern
    Example: P. N. Stern and J. Kerry: Restructuring   66
    Life after Home Loss by Fire
    Dialogue: The Ethics of Interviewing   84

Chapter 5: Dimensional Analysis   86
    Barbara Bowers and Leonard Schatzman
    Example: B. J. Bowers, B. Fibich, & N. Jacobson: 107
    Care as Service, Care as Relating, Care as Comfort:
    Understanding Nursing Home Residents'
    Perceptions of Quality
    Dialogue: Questions?   125

Chapter 6: Shifting the Grounds: 127
    Constructivist Grounded Theory Methods
    Kathy Charmaz

    Example: K. Charmaz, The Body, Identity, and Self: 155
    Adapting to Impairment
    Dialogue: Subjectivity in Analysis   192

Chapter 7: From Grounded Theory to Situational Analysis: 194
    What's New? Why? How?
    Adele E. Clarke

    Dialogue: Questions?   234

Chapter 8: Grounded Theories: On Solid Ground   236
    Janice M. Morse, Adele E. Clarke, Barbara Bowers,
    Kathy Charmaz, Juliet Corbin, and
    Phyllis Noerager Stern

Resources   251

Index   257

About the Authors   263

Dedication

To Anselm and Barney
with gratitude and respect
and to the generations to follow

PREFACE
The Banff Symposium

On September 24, 2007, a one-day symposium, sponsored by the *International Institute for Qualitative Methodology* (IIQM), was held in conjunction with the Advances in Qualitative Methods Conference, in Banff, Alberta. For the first time, the major methodologists of the "second generation"—students of Barney Glaser and Anselm Strauss—gathered to discuss grounded theory, its developments, its controversies, and its forms.

We called it a "Grounded Theory Bash," using *bash* in the celebratory sense. The day met all expectations: more than 200 people attended, and true dialogue centered on grounded theory began. This book arose from that day as a record of the *proceedings* supplemented by additional dialogue with the presenters.

Our intent was to publish the papers as presented at the *Grounded Theory Bash*, along with discussion from the floor that occurred that day. But the book grew beyond that, as, in the months following, the conversations continued as questions arose. We have included some of these later discussions and, to bring some context to the event, introductory and closing chapters were added. In addition, some presenters have included what they consider to exemplary research articles reflecting their "style" of grounded theory, making similarities and differences among the styles more apparent.

Grounded theory is probably the most commonly used qualitative method, surpassing ethnography, and it is used internationally. Unlike ethnography, the developers of grounded theory are clearly identified—Barney Glaser and Anselm Strauss—and their ideas were first published in *Discovery of Grounded Theory* (1967).

Of course, the method did not arise solely from the work of Glaser and Strauss. If we look at previous work in the Chicago School, we see common elements—the *basic social process*, for instance appears in the writing at that time. Although a "new" sociology was emerging from the Chicago School of Sociology, there were no parallel methodological advances to match the theoretical positions of Chicago School sociologists. In the 1960s, qualitative methods books were not readily available, so *Discovery*, plus the active teaching and mentoring of students at UCSF (University of California, San Francisco), created a strong foundation, establishing the "grounded theory school."

Grounded theory has also "taken off" because of other reasons, most notably the mentoring efforts of Glaser and Strauss. The mentoring they provided their students and the collegial team meetings and joint projects they conducted were the envy of doctoral students outside UCSF. Their students developed into a cadre of strong, well-published researchers in their own right, who, in turn, have influenced a new generation of researchers. Their prolific publishing of methods articles and texts, as well as research studies, pushed the method beyond nursing and sociology to all social sciences, and beyond the United States, worldwide, as the numbers of foreign translations of these works attest (see the Resources section).

We dedicate this volume to Anselm and Barney with respect and gratitude. With the exception of Janice Morse, the authors of this book were a part of the cadre of students "hanging around" and over the years, working directly with Anselm and Barney—hence, the *second generation*. They and many other students have contributed directly and indirectly to grounded theory methods. Although our list is not complete, in particular we acknowledge other early students of Glaser and/or Strauss: Barbara Artinian, Jeanne Quint Benoliel, Patrick Biernacki, Carole Chenitz, Eleanor Covan, Elihu Gerson, Shizuko Fagerhaugh, David Maines, Katharyn May, Celia Orona, Susan Leigh Star, Barbara Suczek, Janice Swanson, Carolyn Wiener, and Holly Wilson.

In the spirit of Anselm—for it was his habit to fully acknowledge all contributors as authors in his books—all presenters from the bash are authors of this text. Janice Morse coordinated the session and served as moderator; otherwise, authorship order was allocated in the order that chapters appear in the text. Adele Clarke prepared the Resources section. We thank the University of Alberta's IIQM for their assistance with this effort, and Dori Fortune and Nathan Neilson, University of Utah, and Mitch Allen and Carole Bernard, Left Coast Press, Inc., for their support during production.

We also thank Blackwell Publishers Ltd., *The Gerontologist*, and Wiley-Blackwell Publishing Ltd. for allowing us to reproduce key exemplars of grounded theory in this volume. Those reproduced materials are:

Bowers, B. J., Fibich, B., & Jacobson, N. (2001). Care as service, care as relating, care as comfort: Understanding nursing home residents' perceptions of quality. Reprinted with permission from *The Gerontologist*, 41(4), 539–545.

Charmaz, K. (1995). The body, identity and self. *The Sociological Quarterly*, 36(4), 657–680. Reprinted with permission from Wiley-Blackwell Publishing Ltd., PO Box 805, 9600 Garsington Road, Oxford OX4 2DQ, United Kingdom. All rights reserved.

Stern, P. N. & Kerry, J. (1996). Restructuring life after home loss by fire. Reprinted with permission from *Image, Journal of Nursing Scholarship*, 20(1), 11–16. Copyright, Blackwell Publishers Ltd., reprinted with permission.

Reference

Glaser, B. G. & Strauss, A. L. (1967). *The discovery of grounded theory*. New York: Aldine.

Janice M. Morse
Phyllis Noerager Stern
Juliet Corbin
Barbara Bowers
Kathy Charmaz
Adele E. Clarke

March 2008

1. Tussles, Tensions, and Resolutions

Janice M. Morse

Grounded theory may now be the most commonly used qualitative research method, surpassing ethnography. Despite its relative newness, developed only in 1967, the method is used extensively in North America and internationally. Significantly, this vast expansion has extended from only two researchers, Barnie Glaser and Anslem Strauss, who were at the University of California at San Francisco (UCSF), their students, and their students' students. In four decades, their methods and research publications have created a traceable lineage. What is important is that their method, the majority of which focused on the illness experience and associated phenomena (such as caregiving), has since exploded into other social science disciplines—education, nursing, business, family studies, gerontology, social work, women's and gender studies, cultural studies, and other areas. The influence of grounded theory is now so widespread that it can be argued that it has profoundly changed the face of social science—clearly developing it in several innovative areas.

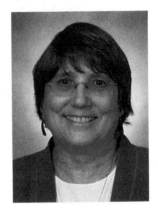

What are these areas? Grounded theory, particularly when used with a symbolic interactionist theoretical lens, enables not only the documentation of change within social groups, but understanding of the core processes central to that change. Grounded theory enables the identification and description of phenomena, their main attributes, and the core, social or social psychological process, as well as their interactions in the trajectory of change. In other words, it allows us to explicate what is *going on* or *what is happening* (or *has happened*) within a setting or around a particular event. But it does even more. It provides us with the tools to synthesize these data, develop concepts, and midrange theory that remains linked to these data, yet is generalizable to other instances and to future instances. Grounded theory is a very powerful tool for the social sciences.

As with all qualitative methods—and with perhaps all research methods—the method cannot be used in a "cookbook" or formulaic way. Every application, every time grounded theory is used, it requires adaptation in particular ways as demanded by the research question, situation, and participants for whom the research is being conducted. But grounded theory is not necessarily a collection of strategies. It is primarily a particular way of thinking about data.

Importantly, this *way of thinking about data* cannot be standardized. When grounded theory is used by researchers from different disciplines, researchers with different personalities and different tolerances for ambiguity, researchers with a varying need for structure, various creative abilities, a knowledge of different social science theory, with various paradigmatic perspectives, research goals, and even individual adherence to and respect for quantitative assumptions and principles, it means that grounded theory is not being *performed* in exactly the same way each time it is used. It means that the end results are not identical in labels, form, or level of abstraction. It means that grounded theories are different to the extent that some researchers use only some of the grounded theory strategies. They may write "methods *approaching* grounded theory were used in this study" (italics added)—and may not be

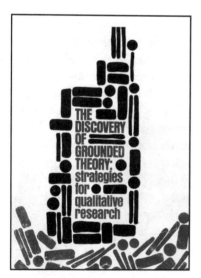

Cover of Glaser, B. G. & Strauss, A. L. (1967). The Discovery of Grounded Theory: Strategies for Qualitative Research. Chicago: Aldine

well understood by many people who say they used it. On the other hand, others may use all of the strategies available and produce exciting, in-depth descriptive or theoretical work.

Thus, we have a situation in which grounded theory varies and has evolved over the years, molded by users of grounded theory. It even changed and evolved as it was used and taught by the two developers of grounded theory—Barney Glaser and Anselm Strauss.

Of course, although they are credited with the development of grounded theory, it did not consist entirely of unique and new techniques—some were already in use by the sociologists of the Chicago School. These sociologists were already writing about social process and conducting fieldwork with the goal of developing theory from these data. But few of these early pioneer researchers were writing methodological texts—even Goffman shunned this task. Thus, the challenge to prepare texts for students and to document how to do research was taken up by Glaser and Strauss, colleagues who had conducted research together for several years. And to them, the time was certainly right to publish their now classic text: *The Discovery of Grounded Theory* (1967).

Tussles: The Emergence of Glaserian and Straussian Grounded Theory

So individualized are the grounded theory approaches to data that almost immediately differences were apparent in the grounded theory strategies conducted by Barney Glaser and Anselm Strauss. These differences were confounded by their different career paths, with Strauss remaining in academia, and Glaser moving onto other endeavors (as described by Phyllis Stern in Chapter 2), until two distinct versions of grounded theory were apparent by the early 1990s. These were identified and labeled by Phyllis Stern as Glaserian and Straussian grounded theory (Stern, 1995). Milestones from this period were Glaser's *Theoretical Sensitivity* (1978) and Strauss's *Qualitative Data Analysis* (1987).

Straussian grounded theory was developed in large part in the collaboration of Anselm Strauss with Juliet Corbin. Julie Corbin observed, dialogued, and collaborated with Anselm over a sixteen-year period, assisting him in explicating what he actually did with data, and assuming a large part of the writing of *Basics of Qualitative Research Analysis* (Strauss & Corbin, 1990). Following Strauss's death, she finalized a second edition in 1998 (Corbin & Strauss, 1998) and has recently written a third (Corbin & Strauss, 2008), which is described in Chapter 3.

Meanwhile, Barney Glaser continued to publish his works through Sociology Press—explicating grounded theory methods, responding to Straussian grounded theory, and publishing collections of grounded theories. He continued to teach grounded theory through workshops and developed a website, mentoring students internationally and serving on their dissertation committees. The development of Glasserian grounded theory is described by Phyllis Stern in Chapter 4.

Resolutions? The Emergence of Other Grounded Theories

The emergence of grounded theory did not stop with the original developers but has continued through their students in a distinct "genealogy" of development (see Figure 1.1).

The first major diversion from grounded theory occurred very early, by Leonard Schatzman, who served a postdoc with Anselm Strauss in the 1950s and joined Strauss at UCSF at his invitation circa 1960. In 1973, again with the intent of producing a text for his students, Schatzman published *Field Research: Strategies for a Natural Sociology* (1973). Coauthored with Strauss, Anselm noted this work was not grounded theory but rather a new method, and *dimensional analysis* emerged. This was further developed in the *Festschrift* in Strauss's honor (Schatzman, 1991), in which Schatzman elaborated its close ties to grounded theory. Barbara Bowers and Leonard Schatzman outline this method in Chapter 5.

Although some students worked intensively with either Barney Glaser or Anselm Strauss, some worked with both. Developing the ideas of both mentors, Kathy Charmaz (2006) developed constructivist grounded theory (see Chapter 6). The last innovation to date is by Adele Clarke, a student of Anselm's who listened to him carefully over the years. She extended grounded theory by incorporating his work on social worlds and arenas and the notion of *situations*. Clarke's *Situational Analysis* (2005) offers techniques to incorporate diverse data sources and embraces the ideas of postmodernism.

Figure 1.1: Genealogy of Grounded Theory: Major Milestones

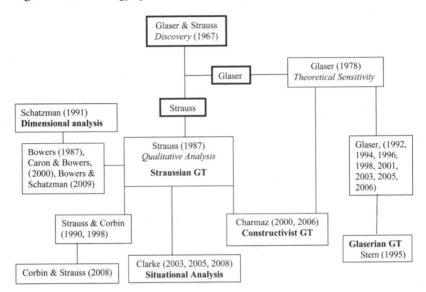

Resolutions?

Science changes, develops, and usually improves over time, and I have no doubt that the methods presented in this book are not the only ones that will emerge. For instance, a considerable literature is developing on the use of computers in analysis, and this is another direction that may change the basic *modus operandi* for doing grounded theory, changing the way grounded theorists *think* and, at the same time, altering the end products—what grounded theory looks like, what it does, and how it is used.

Thus, the present and future emergence of grounded theory introduces a series of interesting questions that must, at some time, be considered:

- If a method is well developed, and that method is published, taught, and used, and that method is changed by a second person, is it still the same method?

- Can research methods be altered and adapted without the permission of the developer?

- Are research methods stable, constant, standardized, or are they individualized according to the topic of the study, differences in participants and settings, and the personality and various knowledge-bases of the users?

- Who has the prerogative to "develop" methods? Expert methodologists or researchers? Doctoral students? Nobody? Anybody? Everybody?

- Or, should there be rules, copyright regulations, and other forms of intellectual property law to protect methods?

Grounded theory evolved and changed—and is still changing. Grounded theory is not a prescribed method that uses a particular "level of data" and formulaic techniques to calculate a solution. Strategies of data gathering and ways of data preparation (coding, categorizing, thematizing) ease the processes of theorizing but by themselves do not make the method. To repeat the mantra one more time: Grounded theory is a way of thinking about data—processes of conceptualization—of theorizing from data, so that the end result is a theory that the scientist produces from data collected by interviewing and observing everyday life.

Let us leave these questions and return to the original purpose of this book—to celebrate grounded theory, to pay our respects to Barney Glaser and Anselm Strauss, and to explore *how* grounded theory has developed throughout the last forty years.

References

Bowers, B. (1987). Intergenerational caregiving: Adult caregivers and their aging parents. *Advances in Nursing Science*, 9(2), 20–31.

Bowers, B. (1994). Dimensional analysis: History and application. Paper presented at the International Nursing Research Conference, Vancouver, BC, Canada, May.

Bowers, B., & L. Schatzman. (2009). *Theory and practice of dimensional analysis: Linking everyday understanding to research methodology*. Walnut Creek, CA: Left Coast Press.

Caron, C., & Bowers, B. (2000). Methods and application of dimensional analysis: A contribution to concept and knowledge development in nursing. In B. L. Rodgers & K. A. Knafl (Eds.), *Concept development in nursing, Foundations, techniques and applications* (pp. 285–319). Philadelphia: W.B. Saunders Co.

Charmaz, K. (2000). Constructivist and objectivist grounded theory. In N. K.

Denzin & Y. S. Lincoln (Eds.), *Handbook of qualitative research,* 2nd ed. (pp. 509–535). Thousand Oaks, CA: Sage.

Charmaz, K. (2006). *Constructing grounded theory.* Thousand Oaks, CA: Sage.

Clarke, A. (2003). Situational analyses: Grounded theory mapping after the postmodern turn. *Symbolic Interaction,* 26(4), 553–576.

Clarke, A. (2005). *Situational analysis: Grounded theory after the postmodern turn.* Thousand Oaks, CA: Sage.

Corbin, J., & Strauss, A. L. (2008). *Basics of qualitative research* (3rd ed.). Thousand Oaks, CA: Sage.

Glaser, B. G. (1978). *Theoretical sensitivity.* Mill Valley, CA: Sociology Press.

Glaser, B. G. (1992). *Emergence versus forcing: Basics of grounded theory analysis.* Mill Valley, CA: Sociology Press.

Glaser, B. G. (1994). *More grounded theory methodology: A reader.* Mill Valley, CA: Sociology Press.

Glaser, B. G. (with the assistance of W. D. Kaplan) (1996). *Gerund grounded theory: The basic social process dissertation.* Mill Valley, CA: Sociology Press.

Glaser, B. G. (1998). *Doing grounded theory: Issues and discussions.* Mill Valley, CA: Sociology Press.

Glaser, B. G. (2001). *The grounded theory perspective: Conceptualization contrasted with description.* Mill Valley, CA: Sociology Press.

Glaser, B. G. (2003). *The grounded theory perspective II: Description's remodeling of grounded theory.* Mill Valley, CA: Sociology Press.

Glaser, B. G. (2005). *The grounded theory perspective III: Theoretical coding.* Mill Valley, CA: Sociology Press.

Glaser, B. G. (2006). *Doing formal grounded theory: A proposal.* Mill Valley, CA: Sociology Press.

Glaser, B. G. & Strauss, A. L. (1967). *The discovery of grounded theory.* New York: Aldine.

Schatzman, L. (1991). Dimensional analysis: Notes on an alternative to the grounding of theory in qualitative research. In D. Maines (Ed.), *Social organization and social process: Essays in honor of Anselm Strauss* (pp. 303–332). New York: Aldine De Gruyter.

Schatzman, L. & Strauss, A. L. (1973). *Field research: Strategies for a natural sociology.* Englewood Cliffs, NJ: Prentice-Hall.

Stern, P. N. (1995). Eroding grounded theory. In J. M. Morse (Ed.), *Critical issues in qualitative research methods* (pp. 212–223). Thousand Oaks, CA: Sage.

Strauss, A. L. (1987). *Qualitative analysis for social scientists.* New York: Cambridge University Press.

Strauss, A. L. & Corbin, J. (1990). *Basics of qualitative research: Grounded theory procedures and techniques.* Newbury Park, CA: Sage.

Strauss, A. L. & Corbin, J. (1998). *Basics of qualitative research: Techniques and procedures for developing grounded theory,* 2nd ed. Newbury Park, CA: Sage.

Dialogue: Doing "Grounded Theory"

Barbara: There are a lot of people who think they know what grounded theory is, but then when they see it actually done, it's quite different than they thought. Many think it is some kind of thematic analysis, some that it's *any* thematic analysis. In the past, when I have been asked to be on a student's committee with faculty who are not grounded theory researchers, the other faculty have been very surprised to see what grounded theory actually is. In some cases, they simply would not agree to let the student use the method. They often said things like "You can use GT but you have to use the same questions for every interview," or "You can use GT but you have to determine your sample in advance, make sure it is representative" or "You can use grounded theory but you must also use random sampling." So when they say, "Yes," giving a student permission to do grounded theory, they're often not saying yes to theoretically sampling—in particular. Sample size is another issue.

They are uncomfortable about not being able to say what step 1 to step 27 will be, what direction you will be going prior to data collection. So, what I have done is let students do a pilot—do two, three interviews, do an analysis, demonstrate the analysis, process and talk about what directions they may be heading based on analysis from the first few interviews, a nice demonstration of the process of grounded theory. And then have the student say where you think you are going to go after that. What I find is other committee members look at that and ask questions, and it's obvious very quickly if it's going to work or not. And I think that's really an important thing to do, because just hearing someone saying "Sure grounded theory is fine" doesn't actually mean it is (fine), and it's a pretty horrible surprise to get half-way down track and then find out that they are not comfortable with it.

The other few things I was going to say is that I think graduate students often have unpredictable and very changeable workloads, especially if they have significant work and family obligations. Grounded theory can't be done by parsing out your time so that you have long lags interspersed with focused work time. And so it doesn't work in my experience when a graduate student says "I'll do my analysis in March and then not get back to it till three months later." You get so far from the data and then people start wanting to take shortcuts and get all the interviews done ahead and write memos later and so forth. It's important to decide whether you are someone who is more comfortable knowing what's coming, where exactly you are going next. I've worked with students and faculty who need to know what's coming next, to have a sense of control in their lives, and to have a high level of predictability; they don't do very well with this method. I've had students who are just furious with me for not saying "Do this and then this," students who are really uncomfortable with the high level of ambiguity that comes with this method and the "false starts" or changing directions—there are a lot of these, exploring different directions and I've had students who have said "But I've wasted my time I went and looked at that and I'm not going to be using it," so I think those are important things to make clear to people and to make them feel okay about it so this is clear from the beginning. But also some students will choose not to do it.

Jan: Kathy do you have anything to add?

Kathy: Well, I found that beginning students, particularly undergraduates, don't want to write memos. They don't want to summarize. They want to go do the analysis, but without doing the requisite analytic work. They want to you to write their memos, even something that would take them say a whole 15 minutes or more!

Adele: I wanted to go back to a point you made earlier, Phyllis, which was when you came to UCSF, you had no family background in higher education, a lack of knowledge of how to go to graduate school, and fear of being found out. And I think that fear of being found out is character-istic of all scholars today who are honest about the inadequacy of our knowledge, 'cause you cannot keep up any more. And many students lack that background. I didn't know you could transfer colleges! But one of the countervailing things that UCSF encourages—and we still really try hard—is to develop among students a very strong cooperative and mutu-ally supportive culture. Then they support each other through gradu-ate school, through their qualitative projects, through their dissertation groups, and throughout their careers. We, in fact, have dinners at the ASA (sociology meetings), to bring alumni and students together and to sustain those kinds of relationships. And I think this comes out of the qualitative research method of working in such small groups that Anselm and Barney sustained. We still do these groups in our courses. I think they sustain all of us, you know, professionals and newbies alike, in trying to produce good work. There is nothing else like it for keeping your mind open.

2. In the Beginning Glaser and Strauss Created Grounded Theory

Phyllis Noerager Stern

I gathered data for this project from my own experience in the doctoral program at the University of California San Francisco (UCSF) from 1973 to 1976, from that of my cohort mate, the gerontologist, Eleanor Krassen Covan, from the World Wide Web, from a chapter Covan and I published in 2001 (Stern & Covan, 2001), from Barney Glaser's response to a questionnaire I e-mailed to him, and from a series of phone calls and e-mails to people who were around at the time.

I start with Glaser and Strauss as real people, as opposed to mythical beings—Anselm Strauss, one of the co-founders of the grounded theory method of research, was born in New York City in 1916 to Jewish immigrants. As a child he developed breathing problems that stayed with him throughout his life—his voice was as soft as his manner. He earned a degree in sociology from the University of Virginia and Master's and doctoral degrees from the University of Chicago. At Chicago, his advisor, Herbert Blumer, a symbolic interactionist (Blumer, 1969), urged him to enroll in a class on social interactionism developed by George Herbert Mead that bore Mead's name even though he had been dead for several years. Because Mead never

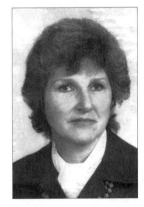

Phyllis Noerager Stern, circa 1980

published, his students published his lecture notes, including a volume edited by Strauss (Mead, 1931/1967). After graduation, Strauss taught at Lawrence College, Indiana University, and the University of Chicago (Online archives of California Anselm L Strauss, 2007). Strauss's next move led to the discovery of grounded theory.

Helen Nahm, then dean of the School of Nursing at UCSF, recruited Anselm Strauss, a well-known sociologist, to the school in 1960. Nahm's purpose was to strengthen the scientific base of the nursing program and to develop the first doctoral program for nurses west of the Mississippi. To this end, Strauss helped develop the Doctor of Nursing Science (DNS) program and later formed the Department of Social and Behavioral Sciences within the School of Nursing. Strauss gathered around him prominent sociologists, Leonard Schatzman and Fred Davis, both alumni of the University of Chicago, and Virginia Olesen, who earned her Master's at the University of Chicago, and her PhD at Stanford. Strauss seized the opportunity to teach nursing students symbolic interactionism. He believed nurses would be less likely to have rigid beliefs about the *received view* of research in the wider world of sociology. To aid the development of the DNS program, Strauss secured a grant entitled "Developing Identities in Nursing," and another grant to study dying in California hospitals. The DNS admitted its first students in 1966 (Flood, 2007). Later, Strauss developed a PhD in sociology, which admitted its first students in 1968. I'm a product of the DNS program, as is Juliet Corbin; Barbara Bowers, Kathy Charmaz, and Adele Clarke graduated from the PhD program in sociology at UCSF.

Barney Glaser was born and raised in San Francisco, California. Glaser earned his undergraduate degree in sociology at Stanford in 1952 then took, according to him, "The natural year abroad after graduation" (Glaser, personal communication, July 26, 2007). He enrolled at the University of Paris, studying literature for the year. In the United States of the 1950s, men were being drafted into the armed services, and Glaser spent two years in the army, one of them in Freiberg, Germany. When Glaser became fluent in German, he took courses in literature at the University of Freiberg (Wikipedia.org/Barney_Glaser, 2007).

At Columbia University, he studied with Paul Lazersfeld and Robert K. Merton, learning descriptive statistics. He earned his PhD in 1961 and then moved back to California. Barney Glaser and Anselm Strauss met "at a gathering," according to Barney (Glaser, personal communication, July 26, 2007). Strauss invited Glaser to join the study on the dying. At this point, Glaser was interested in developing theory. He was well aware of Strauss's reputation as a theoretical sociologist and had read all of Strauss's books. He joined UCSF as a research scientist. The grant on dying lasted four years and generated several publications, the first of which, *Awareness of Dying* (Glaser & Strauss, 1965), had a major impact on the medical community and how dying patients and their families are treated.

Jean Quint (later Benoliel), the first nurse graduate of the DNS program in 1969, was also interested in patients who were dying in hospitals. Glaser and Strauss used some of the data she collected in their *Awareness* book. Glaser and Strauss assumed that because Quint was working on the grant, her data were theirs. Quint assumed otherwise and protested with vigor. She published *The Nurse and the Dying Patient* in 1967 (Quint, 1967), which became a bestseller. The book had a profound effect on nursing education and practice. When I asked her about the incident in 2000, Benoliel said, "Strauss was *always* a gentleman" (Benoliel, personal communication, March 14, 2000), implying, perhaps, that Glaser wasn't. By the time I entered the sociology program, in 1973, Glaser was still defensive about what had happened.

Toward the end of the grant, Glaser and Strauss realized they were using a different method than had been applied to data before—it was ordered, systematic, and marked by rigor. Strauss contributed his experience in theory generation and symbolic interactionism, whereas Glaser's experience with descriptive statistics made it natural for him to visit constant comparisons on the data. Together, they published *The Discovery of Grounded Theory* (Glaser & Strauss, 1967), a book that captured the imagination of social scientists throughout the world. Strauss was already an internationally recognized scholar with several books to his credit and Glaser had published his dissertation research, *Organizational Scientists: Their Professional Careers* (1964); however the two books, *Awareness* (Glaser & Strauss, 1965) and *Discovery* (Glaser & Strauss, 1967) made Barney Glaser's career.

In 1972, Kathy Charmaz attained the first PhD in sociology in UCSF. Adele Clarke graduated in 1985 and did a postdoc at Stanford; Barbara Bowers, a nurse who got her terminal degree in sociology, graduated in 1985; Juliet Corbin earned her DNS in 1981; and I earned mine in 1976.

At thirty-one, Glaser was the new-kid-on-the-block. Strauss was the center of the department, beloved by the other professors. I got the impression that Glaser's success generated a fair amount of resentment in other faculty in the department. For example, after I graduated and joined the faculty of the school of nursing, I offered a small seminar on grounded theory for a few doctoral students. I invited Virginia Olesen to speak to the students. During her stay in the classroom, she ranted about (1) the temerity of a junior faculty member teaching research methods to doctoral students and (2) the invention of new terms for a recognized method, which she called phenomenology, and terms like "core category" and "theoretical codes."

Glaser and Strauss wrote three more books from the study on dying: *Time for Dying* (Glaser & Strauss, 1968), *Anguish: Case Study of a Dying Patient* (Glaser & Strauss, 1970), and *Status Passage* (Glaser & Strauss, 1971), a formal theory. Dying in hospitals was a natural subject for them to study, because as Glaser told me, "both of us had a dying relative experience that was unsatisfactory" (Glaser, personal communication, July 26, 2007).

Glaser offered a course to doctoral students in nursing and sociology, grandly named, "The Discovery of Social Reality," a title that wouldn't wash in this age of reality-depends-on-each-individual's-world-view. He also served on doctoral committees. I think it's important to note that Barney never held a tenure-track position, which explains why he failed to learn which rules of academia one can break and which ones, if broken, earn one a doubtful reputation; interestingly, Marilyn Flood, in her 100-year history of the School of Nursing at UCSF (2007), lists the other sociologists Strauss recruited, but she is silent where Barney Glaser is concerned.

Glaser and Strauss's interpersonal styles were different: Strauss was the consummate mentor whom students and faculty loved and admired. His manner was that of a gentle genius. He had a habit of following a statement with the question, "Get it?" Glaser, on the other hand, covered his vulnerability with abrasiveness; vulnerable because he must have been aware of the coolness of the other faculty in the department. Besides, he earned his PhD in New York City, where one learns defensive skills that may be unnecessary elsewhere. For example, the first day of a class where nurse and sociology students were gathered, he announced that there were too many students and that nurses would need to drop the class. I was desperate, because this was the only method I could see myself doing. When I checked with one of my advisors, Shirley Chater, she told me that the course was under the School of Nursing and it was my *right* to be there (personal communication, 1975). Armed with this new information and figuring I could learn a lot from this guy, I stuck it out.

Now I'm going to add a few words about me as a real person: I spent twenty years working as a three-year diploma nurse. When I had a chance to go for higher degrees, although I got good grades, I felt uncomfortable in the higher educational setting—no one in my extended family finished a baccalaureate degree, my father only attended six years of primary school. For most of my doctoral education, I thought I would be found out—that I didn't really belong in the program. My chair didn't understand the dissertation chapters I submitted to her, and I couldn't seem to convince her that they made sense. This was a powerful woman and head of the department; she gave the impression that she creaked leather, like a cop's gun belt. When I made a tearful phone call to Barney, he suggested I explain to her that this was the way I saw the analysis of the data. When I blubbered, "I can't," Barney responded, "Then I'm through with it—go back to floor nursing." This may sound harsh, but it shocked me back to reality.

In class, Glaser resisted student challenges, but he was open to the analyses of all kinds of data. If he was at times curt, he was equally helpful and clearly expected student success; his take on being a well-read scholar was, "Why read great men, *be* a great man [*sic*]." He took delight in helping students see an obvious path to analysis. We worked through the various processes of grounded theory using one another's data by turns. The products of our cohort impressed the sociology and nursing community (Stern & Covan, 2001). Despite his sometimes egotistical behavior, his protégés regard him as a hero. A *Festchrift* is in the works to honor his long career as a mentor.

Strauss, who had a longstanding heart disease, turned his attention to chronic illness and symbolic interactionism. Glaser and Strauss never again worked as a team, but they remained fast friends.

In 1978, Glaser published, *Theoretical Sensitivity*, his first major book via his own publishing company, to explain the method more clearly. I have found this book helpful and I recommend it to my students. He was putting the book together as my cohort moved through the program. This was before the personal computer, with its cut-and-paste option, was available, and Glaser came to class with lacework notes that had been cut and scotch-taped together. Glaser formed his own publishing company because he believed authors received a pittance for their work, whereas publishers got rich. I believe there is fundamental truth to this view. However, in publishing his own work he skips that most treasured of academic steps—peer review. He didn't understand and still doesn't how dearly we cling to this standard. Nevertheless, he has become his own industry, publishing a book a year and giving workshops all over the world. In 1998, he received an honorary PhD from Stockholm University in Sweden, the highest of academic honors.

From a student's view, it was clear that Glaser and Strauss shared the kind of love that sometimes occurs between mentor and protégé. A rift occurred between the two, occasioned by Strauss's 1990 grounded theory book with Juliet Corbin (Strauss & Corbin, 1990) that Glaser viewed as undermining *his* intellectual property. Glaser published a scathing rejoinder in 1992 attacking the book, chapter by chapter. He reacted as Virginia Olesen had to the language of grounded theory. The wounds soon healed, however, such was their love for one another, and Barney Glaser continues to dedicate his books to Anselm. In all, Barney has published thirteen books and readers through Sociology Press. His new research partner, Judith A. Holton, edits the on-line journal *Grounded Theory Review*, published by Sociology Press.

Strauss died in 1996, but his and Glaser's gift to research, grounded theory, lives on. I'm eternally grateful to them for developing an avenue where I can express my creative talents and describe social scenes as I see them through the collection and analysis of data and the art that is research.

References

Blumer, H. (1969). *Symbolic interactionism*. Berkeley: University of California Press.

Flood, M. E. (2007). *Promise on Parnassus: The first century of the UCSF School of Nursing*. San Francisco: UCSF School of Nursing Press.

Glaser, B. G. (1964). *Organizational scientists: Their professional careers*. Indianapolis: Bobbs-Merrill.

Glaser, B. G. (1978). *Theoretical sensitivity*. Mill Valley, CA: Sociology Press.

Glaser, B. G. (1992). *Basics of grounded theory analysis*. Mill Valley: Sociology Press.

Glaser, B. G. & Strauss, A. L. (1965). *The awareness of dying*. Chicago: Aldine.

Glaser, B. G. & Strauss, A. L. (1967). *The discovery of grounded theory*. Chicago: Aldine. Glaser, B. G. & Strauss, A. L. (1968). *Time for dying*. Chicago: Aldine.

Glaser, B. G. & Strauss, A. L. (1970). *Anguish: Case study of a dying patient*. Chicago: Aldine

Glaser, B. G. & Strauss, A. L. (1971). *Status passage: A formal theory*. Chicago: Aldine.

Mead, G. H. (1967). *On social psychology: Selected papers* (A. L. Strauss, Ed.). Chicago: University of Chicago Press. (Original lectures written in 1931.)

Online archives of California Anselm L. Strauss. (2007). The Regents of the University of California. Available online at http://www.ucsf.edu/anselmstrauss/ (accessed July 26, 2007.)

Quint, J. (1967). *The nurse and the dying patient*. New York: Macmillan.Stern, P. N. & Covan, E. K. (2001). Early grounded theory: Its processes and products. In R. S. Schreiber & P. N. Stern (Eds.), *Grounded theory in nursing* (pp. 17–34). New York: Springer.

Strauss, A. L. & Corbin, J. (1990). *Basics of qualitative research: Grounded theory procedures and techniques*. Newbury Park, CA: Sage.

www.Wikipedia.org/Barney Glaser. Accessed July 28, 2007.

Photo Album

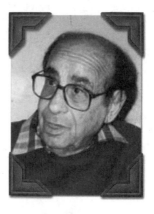

2.1: *Professor Anselm Strauss (deceased)*
(Photo from the informal archives of the Department of Social and Behavioral Sciences, UCSF)

2.2: *Solomon Davis (deceased) talking to Barney Glaser, circa 1988*
(Photo from the informal archives of the Department of Social and Behavioral Sciences, UCSF)

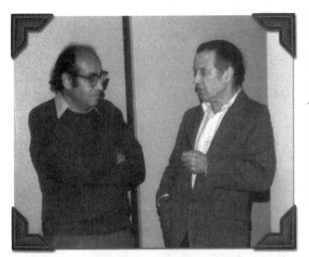

2.3: Anselm Strauss (left) talking to Lenny Schatzman at a baby shower for Barbara Bowers, 1983. (Photo from the informal archives of the Department of Social and Behavioral Sciences, UCSF)

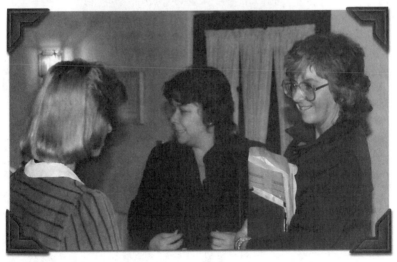

2.4: Lynda Derugin, staff MSO (business officer) talking to Adele Clarke (center) and Kathy Charmaz (right) at the 20th birthday party of the Doctoral Sociology Program, circa 1988

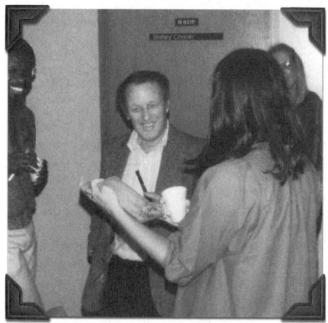

2.5: Leonard Schatzman (Photo from the informal archives of the Department of Social and Behavioral Sciences, UCSF)

2.6: Anselm Strauss (d. 1996) and Julie Corbin in a research session, circa 1990 (Photo Julie Corbin)

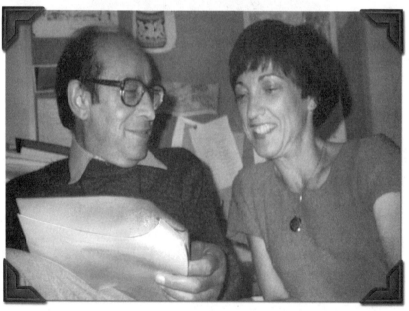

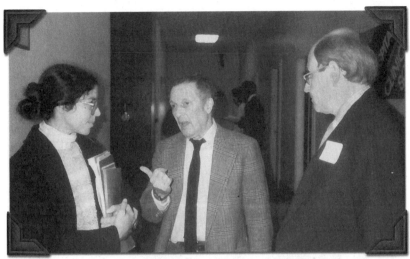

2.7: Left to right: Professor Nancy Adler (UCSF Dept. of Psychiatry), Professor Emeritus Lenny Schatzman, and Marty Prosono (PhD UCSF)

(Photo from the informal archives of the Department of Social and Behavioral Sciences, UCSF)

2.8: Leonard Schatzman

(Photo from the informal archives of the Department of Social and Behavioral Sciences, UCSF)

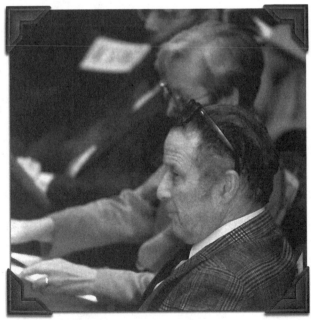

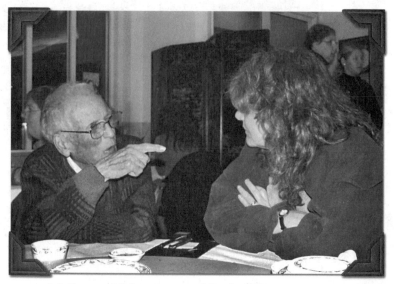

2.9: Leonard Schatzman and Barbara Bowers
(Photo Barbara Bowers)

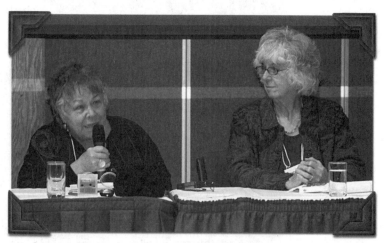

2.10: Adele Clarke and Kathy Charmaz, circa 2007
(Photo courtesy of Mary Barros-Bailey, Boise, ID)

3. Taking an Analytic Journey

Juliet Corbin

O ver the last ten to fifteen years, many new ideas have emerged regarding qualitative research. These ideas have had a considerable impact on me as a professional. Although I was asked to write about Strauss's version of grounded theory, I find that I can no longer write about what is strictly Strauss's version. Too much time has elapsed since Anselm Strauss has died, and to write about his version implies that over time and with usage a methodology does not undergo change. It also implies that the people who write and talk about that method are not subject to change. Therefore, though in this chapter I have tried to be true to Strauss's version of the methodology, there remains the possibility that what I am about to write reflects as much my present interpretation as it does his original thoughts about method. In fact anyone who writes about a research method, other than the original author, is writing about his or her interpretation of that method because it is method as filtered through the eyes of that second person. That is why I felt it necessary to spend some time early in this chapter explaining how I've changed in response to contemporary thought in the field of qualitative research. Furthermore, in this chapter I wanted to do more than just talk about method, I wanted to illustrate how it is

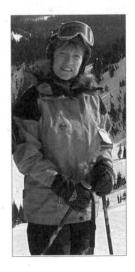

done using an example from *Basics of Qualitative Research*, 3rd edition (Corbin & Strauss, 2008). I conclude the chapter with a discussion of what I believe Strauss's version of grounded theory has to offer researchers.

People Change and Methods Change

My first encounter with qualitative research began in what I call the "Age of the Dinosaurs." In those days, I was a naive Master's student taking the required research course. I found the quantitative part of the class pretty dry. It didn't stimulate my interest for doing research. However, when the class presentation turned to a discussion of qualitative research methods, I said, "What is this? Tell me more." There was something about qualitative research that I found very appealing, though at the time I couldn't have told you what that was. Looking back, I believe that qualitative research resonated with me then and continues to do so because it touches at the heart of what nursing is all about: reaching out to people, listening to what they have to say, and then using that knowledge to make a difference in their lives.

When it came time to do a Master's thesis, my advisors strongly suggested that I do a quantitative study because there was no one in the department sufficiently trained in qualitative methods to guide me through the process. Even before completing the Master's degree, I decided that I wanted to go on for a doctorate at the University of California in San Francisco (UCSF) and, once there, learn to do qualitative research. At UCSF, I discovered many able mentors. Among them were Ramona Mercer, Phyllis Stern, Leonard Schatzman, and Anselm Strauss. Little did I know when I began my doctoral program that I would end up doing research and writing books with Anselm Strauss, least of all a book about his research methodology.

Before discussing how I've changed over the years, I want to provide some background regarding the state of qualitative research at the time that I began my doctoral program in 1976. I want to review that history briefly because of the influence it had on the writing of earlier editions of *Basics* (Strauss & Corbin, 1990, 1998) and the method presented in that text.

In the old days, it was not unusual to hear ideas such as:

1. Theory is embedded in the data. The idea was that if the researcher is sensitive and looks and hard enough at the data, theory will emerge, the key word being "emergence."

2. A researcher should remain "objective" at least to some degree when collecting and analyzing data.

3. At all cost, a researcher should avoid "going native" (adopting the stance of or getting too close to participants), because going native would make it difficult to maintain that objectivity.

4. Though it was acknowledged that there was no "one" truth, there was still the notion that a research could capture a semblance of "reality" in data and present that reality as a set of theoretical findings.

Today, these ideas seem outdated, but I mention them to make a point. As with any phenomena, they have to be located within the context of time and place. When the first edition of *Basics* was published, many of us (the collective us) adopted the then prevailing notions about qualitative research. But, methodology is a living thing in the sense that it has to be given credit for the possessing the possibility of change. Here, change doesn't mean that the philosophical underpinnings of Strauss's version of grounded theory have been abandoned. The method remains rooted in pragmatism and symbolic interactionism, with its emphasis on structure and process. What has changed is subtle and has to do with how I approach, think, and write about qualitative research. With time, some researchers have simply walked away from the more traditional approaches to doing qualitative research, some going so far as to blur the boundaries between fiction and research. Others, like me, have tried to hold on to what is good about the past while updating a method to bring it more in line with the present.

In writing the third edition of *Basics of Grounded Theory* (Corbin & Strauss, 2008), I have chosen parts of both past and present and rejected others. I think I have retained what was best about Strauss's approach to doing analysis. One must remember that each research project is different, and that each person using a methodology, even with different projects, infuses the method with some aspect of the self and of the project and in doing so changes that methodology somewhat to make it more relevant. If Anselm Strauss were alive today, it is more than likely he would have changed also for he never stood still. I admire the works of Clarke (2005) and Charmaz (2006) and how they've applied postmodernist and constructivist paradigms to grounded theory methodology, taking up the challenge of Denzin (1994) to move interpretative methods more deeply into the regions of postmodern sensibility (p. 512).

The first edition of *Basics* was written mostly as a text for us to use with our own students. Strauss and I never thought that it would become a popular text or that it would create any controversy. We simply wanted to provide our students with a handy guide that they could refer back to once they left the security of the classroom to go out on their own and work on their dissertations. Because the book retained its popularity over the years, despite the publication of other texts on qualitative analysis, Strauss and I were asked to write the second edition of *Basics*. Unfortunately, Anselm Strauss died before that edition was completed. In keeping with Anselm's memory and the popular nature of the book, I felt it best not to make too many changes at the time. Eventually, I was asked to write a third edition of *Basics*.

The challenge I faced when writing that third edition was how to hold on to what is best about Strauss's basic approach to doing analysis, while bringing his methodology more in line with contemporary thought and the changes that had taken place within myself. I had no simple term to classify the person I'd become methodologically over the years since Dr. Strauss's death. I realized that, like him, I was a mixture of many philosophical orientations. The pragmatist/interactionist perspective that influenced Strauss so deeply is also an essential part of who I am, and, therefore, the method I present in the third edition of *Basics*. But there is more. As Denzin (1998) says so well when talking about qualitative research today: "Clearly simplistic classifications do not work. Any given qualitative researcher-as-bricoleur can be more than one thing at the same time, can be fitted into both the tender-and the tough-minded categories" (p. 338). More specifically, below are some of the contemporary ideas about qualitative researcher that I've adopted and built into the third edition of *Basics* (2008).

There is not one reality; there are multiple "realities," and collecting and analyzing data require capturing and taking into account those multiple viewpoints. There may be external events, such as a full moon, a war, and an airplane crashing into a building, but these are not themselves as important as how persons experience these events and respond to them. As Schawndt (1998) states: "One can reasonably hold that concepts and ideas are invented (rather than discovered) yet maintain that these inventions correspond to something in the real world" (p. 237). Therefore, it is not events themselves that are the focus of our studies but the meanings given to events and the actions/interactions/emotions expressed in response, along with the context in which those responses and the events occur.

Each person experiences, gives meaning to, and responds to events in light of his or her own biography or experiences, according to gender, time and place, cultural, political, religious, and professional backgrounds. To see the validity of this statement, one only has to turn on the television and listen to a group of people discussing an event, such as a political speech. There is much discourse and sometimes outright conflict about what was said, but there is rarely total agreement about the significance or even content of the event. What a viewer sees and hears are multiple viewpoints on the same topic (but this doesn't mean that there are no patterns of response). Add to this the notion that what is being seen and heard on the television is filtered through the viewer's interpretation of the event based on his or her personal history and biography and you get a very complicated picture, one that can never be fully understood or reconstructed by the researcher.

I agree with the constructionist viewpoint that concepts and theories are constructed (they don't emerge) by researchers out of stories that are told by research participants who are trying to explain and make sense out of their experiences and/or lives, both to the researcher and themselves. Out of these multiple constructions, analysts build something that they call knowledge. Schawndt (1998) says:

> In a fairly unremarkable sense, we are all constructivists if we believe that the mind is active in the construction of knowledge. Most of us would agree that knowing is not passive—a simple imprinting of sense data on the mind—but active; mind does something with these impressions, at the very least forms abstractions of concepts. In this sense, constructivism means that human beings do not find or discover knowledge so much as construct or make it. We invent concepts, models, and schemes to make sense of experience and further we continually test and modify these constructions in light of new experience. (p. 237)

Perhaps it is the nurse in me who is talking because, although I realize that knowledge is constantly evolving in light of new experience and findings are "constructions" and not exact replicas of reality, I believe that both doing "interpretive" work and conceptualizing data are necessary because it is necessary to have a language to talk about the phenomena and problems encountered by practitioners in any field. As Blumer (1969) states, without a conceptual language there is no basis for discussion, conflict, negotiation, or development of a knowledge-based practice. We can't have practitioners walking around doing things without having a body of theoretical knowledge, along with their experience, to guide their actions. Knowledge may not mirror reality, but it does help us understand human response.

I am practical in what I want to accomplish with my research. Like Anselm, I draw on pragmatists and interactionists such as Blumer (1969), Hughes (1971), Park (1967), Thomas (1966), and their vision of research as the foundation for bringing about change. I agree with the social justice aims of feminist research (Oleson, 1998). At the same time, I enjoy doing qualitative research for research's sake—the people I meet, the intellectual stimulation I receive, and the opportunity to make order out of disorder. I agree with the feminist notion that we don't separate who we are as persons from the research and analysis that we do. Therefore, we must be self-reflective about how we influence the research process and, in turn, how it influences us. Hamberg and Johansson (1999) explain what they did to be self-reflective, and I, too, try to carry this out in my research. They say:

> For this reflexive analysis, we have reread the coded interviews to scrutinize parts featuring tension, contradictions, or conflicting codes—passages that had often been discussed when we were striving to find reasonable and legitimate interpretations. We have also read our memos to recall our instant reactions during, and after, the interviews and our discussions when we compared our coding. (p. 458)

Though readers of research construct their own interpretations of findings, the fact that these are constructions and reconstructions does not negate the relevance of the findings or the insights that can be gained from them. I believe that we share a common culture out of which common constructions or agreements about the meaning of concepts can be arrived at through discourse. Concepts give us a basis for discourse and arriving at shared understandings. Therefore, I will continue to believe in the power of concepts and advocate their use.

There is another point that I believe is important to make here because there have been some misunderstandings about how Strauss and I use techniques and procedures. Techniques and procedures are tools to be used by the researcher as he or she sees fit to solve methodological problems. They are not a set of directives to be rigidly adhered to. No researcher should become so obsessed with following a set of coding procedures that the fluid and dynamic nature of qualitative analysis is lost. The analytic process is first and foremost a thinking process. It requires stepping into the shoes of the other and trying to see the world from their perspective. Analysis should be relaxed, flexible, and driven by insight gained through interaction with data rather than being structured and based on procedures.

Following through on the Challenge

As I worked on the third edition of *Basics*, I struggled with how to put together the best of the past with what I believe about research in the present. All sorts of questions formed in my mind as I sat down to write: What are methods? Are they merely sets of procedures? Or are they philosophical approaches with few if any procedures? What role do methods play in research? Are they guides, or just a broad set of ideas? What and how much instructional structure is necessary is necessary to guide readers through the process? What is the role of the researcher? How do you acknowledge the researcher while still telling the story of participants? How much or how little interpretation should be involved?

In addition to the above questions, there were several other broad issues complicating the writing of the third edition of *Basics*. Since the original publication of *The Discovery of Grounded Theory* (Glaser & Strauss, 1967), many different approaches to doing grounded theory have emerged, leaving me to wonder *if there is* or *even should be* a method called "grounded theory." Perhaps it would be better to think of grounded theory as a copendium of different methods that have as their purpose the construction of theory from data, with each version of grounded theory method having its own philosophical foundation and approach to data gathering and analysis, while sharing some common procedures. Then there is the even larger question: Is theory-constructing research still relevant today? If there is not one but multiple "realities" out there, is it possible or even practical to package findings into one theoretical explanatory scheme, while acknowledging that any theory is limited in its explanatory ability? Wouldn't thick rich description, case analysis, change directed research, or telling stories provide more valid reasons for doing research?

I was rather daunted by the task in front of me in writing the third edition. I procrastinated, wrote, and rewrote as one does when trying on ideas. But once I got into the "groove" of writing I found myself enjoying the process. I discovered that I wasn't delineating a whole new method. I was modernizing the method I had grown up with, dropping a lot of the dogma, flexing up procedures, and even seeking ways to explain how computers might enhance the research process.

The Method

As I stated in the introduction of this chapter, what I'm getting at in this long discussion is that it is impossible for me, from the perspective of the person I've become, to talk about methodology in the way that I did ten or fifteen years ago. I can't say this is Strauss's version of grounded theory because how I talk about method in the present (and how I've written about it in the third edition of *Basics*) is a combination of:

- what I felt was best about Strauss's method;

- combined with what I've derived from contemporary thought;

- all seen through the perspective of the person I've become over the years based on readings, continued research and life experiences, and interactions with students both in teaching methods in various parts of the world and over the Internet.

Therefore, rather than going into an entire philosophical or method-ological discussion about "Straussian" grounded theory, I want to present an example of how I would go about doing research today based on every-thing that I presented above. The example is taken from the third edition of *Basics*. What I hope to convey with this example is that though the essentials of Strauss's method remains, I have become much more fluid and open when doing analysis. I use all the procedures, but they remain in the background rather than looming in the foreground. Bear with me as I describe the most recent and most satisfying piece of research of my entire career: a study of participants in the Vietnam War. Now this topic doesn't sound much like nursing, but it does have implications for the delivery of nursing care to young soldiers who participate in wars and is especially relevant in light of present events.

After I completed the introductory chapters of the third edition of *Basics*, I thought about how to best demonstrate to students the fluid and dynamic nature of data collection and analysis. I wanted to emphasize the interaction that occurs between the researcher and the data and to demonstrate how it is a combination of the data and the researcher's interpretation of them that guides and stimulates the ongoing research process. The usual way that authors do this is to present excerpts from their previous studies. But I wanted to do a research project right in front of my readers, take them through the process from beginning to end. Furthermore, I wanted to study something that I had never studied before. I wanted readers to see the methodological problems that I encountered along the way, to see how I handled these, and to obtain some insight into what I was thinking while doing the research. I wanted to share my experience. Stated more plainly, I wanted to demonstrate how to blend the best of contemporary thought with what was good about past approaches to doing research.

At the time, I didn't realize how long it would take me to do a research project as part of a book about methodology. Or how involved I would become with the subject matter. Even though I had an idea of what I wanted to do methodologically, I didn't have a topic for the research. I began looking through my files and found an interview done by Dr. Strauss some years ago with one of my close friends about his experiences as a nurse during the Vietnam War. After perusing that interview, I knew that I had found the topic for my study—the Vietnam War. I had grown up during the Vietnam era yet knew little about that event. This was an opportunity to inform myself as well as to demonstrate to readers of my book how to analyze data. I want to make clear that it is very important for a researcher to be excited about the topic he or she is studying. It is difficult for a researcher to be creative, do the hard work required, and keep plodding along over time if she or he lacks a passion for what is being studied.

Note that I had no specific research question when I began the analysis. I wasn't sure where I was going with the research. I was just going to sit down with that first piece of data in front of me and let it flow, let the research take me where it wanted. To bring my readers along with me, I wrote my thoughts down in a series of memos, but these are too lengthy to replicate here so I'll describe the process and some of my findings.

Analytic Process

The way that I analyzed the data was to break them apart into pieces corresponding to natural breaks in the flow of conversation. Then I worked with that piece of data. I sought to identify what I thought participants were telling me. I tried out various interpretations and discarded those that were not supported by data. I used concepts to capture my interpretations. I compared various pieces of data within and between participants looking for similarities and differences. Once I had some concepts, I scrutinized the data for descriptors or qualifiers of those concepts. In other words, I looked for properties of concepts and how they varied dimensionally.

Let me give an example. Participant #1 began the interview by explaining something about himself before going to war. He went on to say a little about why he decided to volunteer as an army nurse. I conceptualized this description as the "prewar self." Some of the properties of his prewar self were youth, idealism, a sense of patriotism, innocence about war, training as a nurse, and having a family that supported the war and his joining the military.

The significance of the concept "prewar self" meant little to me early in the analysis. It just seemed important at the time to write a memo describing the characteristics of the men and women before they went to Vietnam. I knew that each person would be different in the details but that each person I interviewed would have a prewar self.

One major point about qualitative research in this manner is that in the beginning of the analysis, the researcher doesn't know with any certainty the degree of significance of early concepts. The researcher just kind of knows intuitively that something is important and should be noted. For example, though I realized that it was important to know something about who a person was before going off to war, it was not until I got deeper into the analysis that I discovered that the concept the "prewar self" was part of higher level concept (or category) I termed the "changing self." I made this discovery by noting that the manner in which women and men described themselves before *going* to war was considerably different from how they described themselves *during* their time in Vietnam and how they described themselves *after* leaving Vietnam.

I derived many concepts while coding this first interview. However, it wasn't until I was almost finished analyzing the first interview that two things struck me as especially noteworthy. I noticed that this man described his "experience" in Vietnam as being "not so bad." In fact, he described it as a "very maturing" experience. This struck me as rather odd, because I came of age during the Vietnam era and everything I read or saw on TV at the time made me think that going to war was a "terrible" experience. (I later learned that an experience can be difficult or even terrible and still be maturing.)

Drawing on my background knowledge, I asked myself how it could be that this man's experience was not so bad. In doing so, I was picking up the not-so-bad dimension of the experience. I thought about this descriptor for a while and came to suspect that participant #1's experience was not so bad because he was a nurse, a noncombatant. Although he flew in helicopters into war zones to pick the injured, he never had to engage in battle or kill enemy soldiers. The other thing that struck me about the interview was that although it was never overtly expressed, there seemed to be a lot of residual anger and ambivalence about the war experience and how the war was handled. And most revealing to me was that participant #1 said in the interview that he had *never* spoken to another person about his experiences in Vietnam. Although his two brothers and many of his friends had also served in Vietnam, his talking to Dr. Strauss was the first time he had ever revealed anything about his experience there. I later learned that "not talking about Vietnam" was a common theme among Vietnam veterans. They essentially wall off that part of their life.

I mulled those thoughts over for a while and came up with two questions that would guide the next steps of the research. The first question was: Would the war experience be different for "combatants," that is, persons who went to Vietnam and participated in combat? And, the second question: Why is there still the wall of silence and so much residual anger? These questions guided the next steps in my data collection and analysis. I was doing theoretical sampling or directing data collection on the basis of the concepts "combatant" and "noncombatant," "wall of silence," and "residual anger." In addition to specifically looking for data that would bring out these concepts, I would examine subsequent data in terms of the "prewar self" and other concepts derived from that first analysis of data.

At this early stage of the research, I couldn't be certain that I was going in the right direction with the research. I had to trust my instincts. I let my interpretation of what I perceived to be significant guide me to the next phase of research. I still didn't have a well-formulated overall research question. I didn't know exactly what I was looking for. Up to this point in my research career, I had never trusted my own intuitive responses to data to such an extent. Usually I had some vague research question in mind when I began a research project. This time, rather than a specific question directing the research from the onset, the questions that evolved during my interaction with the data shaped the direction the research would take.

I was ready to move on with the study, following up on the concepts of "combatant" versus "noncombatant," when I realized I didn't have another participant to interview. I didn't know anyone who had been a combatant in the Vietnam War. My next methodological problem was to figure out where I could I find a group of Vietnam War combatants to interview. I turned to the Internet, where so many people go these days for help, and put out a request for participants. *Oh my, what a discovery that was!* After several days, I received a reply to my request. I mean just *one* response, whereas I had expected to be overloaded with willing participants. The responder, a Vietnam veteran stated that he would be happy to answer my questions about his time in Vietnam. He was willing to talk because he was interested in educating people about the Vietnam War. However, he wanted to warn me that I shouldn't expect a response from other veterans because even though thirty years had passed since the war, many vets were still having difficulty coping with their experience in Vietnam. I was rather astounded that the Vietnam War was still causing so much suffering.

I did receive another e-mail from someone in the same chat group. It said, "If I can't even tell my wife about the war, what makes you think I can talk to you." Ouch. I thought at this point that maybe it was not such a good idea to do a study on Vietnam War veterans. Eventually, I did get another response and the third responder was willing to talk about his experience. I had two more participants for my study and felt that I could continue with the analysis begun months earlier.

I asked Participant #2 what it was like to be a combatant. I wanted to compare the first two interviews for similarities and differences. I still had no general question in mind or sense of where I was going with the study, but I was pushing forward. Participant #2 was not overly verbose but what he said was quite startling, at least to me. At first, I wasn't certain that I should put his interview in my book. I was concerned that readers might be frightened by such graphic words about war. Participant #2 told me that war is about killing. You kill the enemy before he kills you. He also said that although a soldier goes into war with sense of idealism and patriotism, these virtues become lost at the time of the first battle. When you are in a war zone being shot at day after day, it all comes down to survival—your own and the survival of your marine brothers.

Then I asked him about the anger. He said there were several things that made him angry. The first thing was that the Americans lost the war, the first war they had ever lost. He believed that the hands of those who actually did the fighting in the war were constrained by the many rules of engagement put on them by the policymakers in Washington. Second, he said that he was angry because 58,000 men lost their lives in a war that had no purpose. Third, he was angry because of the reception veterans received on their homecoming. The arguments about whether the Vietnam War was a just war didn't filter down to the combatants in the field. They believed they were fighting for their country. Moreover, combatants can't easily leave the war behind just because they leave the battlefield and return home. They bring the war home with them in the form of memories and nightmares.

After analyzing interview #2, I knew that I had to learn more about the "war experience" per se and about "survival," two new major concepts. I realized something occurred during combat that made the difference between how combatants versus noncombatants experienced the war.

At this point, the research project began to take on a life of its own outside of the book on methodology that I was writing. I had been touched by the stories that I heard and as a researcher I was emotionally invested in retelling that story. At the same time, I realized that I couldn't become too emotionally invested or I would not be able to complete the book. I also realized that this research would require a lot more investigative work because there were still so many unanswered questions. I was a little frightened because I still wasn't sure where I was going with this research. I would have to continue to trust in myself and in the research process.

I turned to the interview with Participant #3, the only other veteran who responded to my request for participants. I wanted to explore with him the concept of "anger" in greater depth. I wondered if he had a different explanation for why anger seemed so much a part of each of these interviews. Could he explain why, after all these years, so many vets have not let go of the anger and "healed."

Participant #3 told me that the anger begins in boot camp where the drill instructors demean you and wear you down. The purpose of their tactics, from his perspective, was to generate anger, and thereby turn raw recruits into a team that sticks together and that sees the outsider as an enemy. Then, once a soldier gets to war, the anger increases because a soldier realizes that he or she is simply being shot at because they are there: "You don't even know the people who are shooting at you." If you are lucky enough to survive the experience and return home, you then discover that those who remained at home were going on with their lives as usual. They went to college, got married, and had good jobs. The vets thought that family, friends, and non-vets just couldn't relate to what a combatant has been through, nor could they understand the nightmares and the difficulties of readjustment to civilian life.

With the analysis of three interviews behind me, I still had many more questions about the research than I had answered. I didn't know much about the actual experience of combat. Furthermore, I needed to put the war experience into a larger historical and political context to better understand it. I realized that I would have to know more about the rules of engagement and the policies that brought the United States and Vietnam into war. I also needed to know more about this enemy, the North Vietnamese and the Viet Cong, and why they fought so fiercely. I needed to examine combat situations and analyze them so that I could understand more about the process of surviving and why, although 58,000 men died (a large number), many more survived to return home.

Because I had no more participants, I wondered how I was going to acquire that data. I turned to the Internet once more, this time going to Amazon.com. Here I made interesting discovery. Though the Vietnam veterans in the chat room I connected with had difficulty talking about the war, apparently there were many other veterans who were willing to put their stories in print. I had found a fountain of data in the form of *memoirs*. I ordered as many books as I could from Amazon, some written by combatants, others written by nurses, helicopter, and fighter pilots, and some written by prisoners of war and journalists. I even found a couple of books written by Viet Cong soldiers, because in qualitative research it is important to get those multiple perspectives. I also ordered several historical books about the war and about Vietnam to find data about *contextual questions*, like the events that led up to this war; further, I read about the profiles of the men in Washington who directed the war from afar and set the rules of engagement. Their perspective was important, too.

I soon found myself overloaded with data. I learned more about war than I ever wanted to know. I had trouble sleeping. I became stressed every time I looked at the materials. I decided that I needed to distance myself from these war materials for a while so that I could return and do a proper analysis.

When I did return to the study, I analyzed the memoirs in the same way as I did the interviews. I built on the concepts and questions derived from each previous analysis continuing on with theoretical sampling. In the memoirs, I discovered that surviving in war is situational and proportional to the risks associated with those situations. I learned that the greatest death rates occurred in men inexperienced with war and that survival is enhanced when one becomes "a seasoned soldier." However, with time and exposure to conflict, even seasoned soldiers tend to "wear down," which, in turn, increases their chances of being killed or wounded. I discovered that the men fighting the war saw it as war that seemed to go nowhere. There was not attempt to gain or hold territory. Rather, success was based on body counts. The soldiers would fight the enemy and take over a piece of territory only to walk away after the battle, leaving the enemy free to retake that territory. When pushed, the enemy would retreat above 17th parallel, the division line between North and South Vietnam or go into Cambodia or Laos, also supposedly out of bounds according to the rules of engagement. There was a high mortality and morbidity rate on both sides, though the main concern for U.S. soldiers was for their own lost comrades. Then, especially relevant for the soldiers, was the lack of support for the war at home, which was demoralizing.

Most soldiers served their country with honor. But a few soldiers committed atrocities, and often it was the atrocities and not the good things that soldiers did that made the news. Some atrocities occurred because soldiers were worn down by the stress of continuously being in a war zone and not knowing who among the civilian population was enemy and who was friend. As a consequence, combatants sometimes fired at anyone who acted suspicious. This is understandable, as the enemy sometimes hid within civilian populations. I am not excusing soldiers' bad behavior because some were just bad people who happened to be in the military. Others were young, easily influenced, and lacking in adequate leadership, officers to monitor their behavior, and set moral standards. Sometimes soldiers were just plain angry about seeing a comrade die before their eyes and wanted to revenge their comrade's death by punishing the enemy or, worse, hurting civilians who got in the way. But anger also had a positive side in that it could also keep some soldiers alive, contributing to their survival even when they were fatigued and disillusioned with war. The problem was not being able to let go of that anger once soldiers returned home and to civilian life.

These findings led me to another question and more theoretical sampling. If the risks of wearing down were so high, I wondered why some men were able to physically survive and at the same time maintain their moral integrity. Why is it that despite the terrible things that occur in any war, there are also heroes and men and women who did very good deeds for civilian populations? I turned to the data to look at specific situations of risks and analyzed them. I looked at the personal and social psychological conditions that enable soldiers to survive and overcome the physical, psychological, and moral risks associated with war. Later I examined the data to determine why some individuals were able to heal after the war whereas others suffered from posttraumatic stress disorder. What I discovered was that to survive physically and psychologically, combatants had to be able to put aside their prewar civilian selves, adjust to the "realities of war," then, when they returned home, readjust once again by constantly shifting their images of "self" and the "meanings of war." I termed the ability to make these transitions "surviving: reconciling multiple realities," and it became the core concept of my study. The study was more complicated than this, but this gives you some idea of how I proceeded with the study and why I went in the directions that I did.

I won't bore you with all of the details of that study. Anyone interested in learning more about this research can look at the third edition of *Basics*. I want to emphasize that although in methodology texts we talk about procedures, these analytic techniques are just broad guidelines that are used in a very dynamic and flexible ways to stimulate the analysis. Whenever a writer tries to put into words what he or she does when doing analytic work, it becomes rigidified and open to unintended uses. Yet, the actual research process is fluid, dynamic, and evolving. Notice that I had no idea in the study presented above of where I was going at the beginning of the study. I let my interpretations in the form of concepts and the questions I asked about those concepts guide each step of the research process. Throughout the analysis, I felt like a detective following up on one lead after another until I could piece together a whole story. I marveled at the information that a researcher can obtain from data if he or she asks the right questions and takes the time to write memos. In memos, it's not just the researcher and not just the data that are talking, but a combination of researcher and the data interacting together to come up with an explanation of what is going on. Memos are a reflection, the records of that interaction. There is no possibility of omitting the writing of memos as a way of shortcutting the research process. In the end, not having those memos to refer back to shows up in the quality of the product that is produced. The density and variation are missing from the final product because there is no way that a researcher can remember all the details of the analysis.

Concluding Remarks

I think that anyone picking up the third edition of *Basics* will find that in many ways it is a different book from the first and second editions, while at the same time it retains much of the essential elements of Anselm Strauss's approach to developing grounded theory. I think it takes the best of the past and puts it together with contemporary thought to present a method that can lead to the development of "quality" qualitative research. This approach to qualitative research analysis encourages researchers to enter the investigation with an open mind, ready to hear what participants are saying, and advocates letting the questions that emerge from analysis guide the next steps in data collection and analysis. It is a method that rejects a dogmatic and rigid approach to doing research and embraces taking the role of the other, giving voice to participants, all the while noting how the researcher him- or herself is responding and shaping the research.

The researcher formulates new questions as the research evolves, chooses among a variety of data sources and analytic strategies, and even changes the course of the research midway as the situation demands. As in other qualitative research, the self is the instrument of the research. It requires that a researcher trust his or her instincts about where to go, what kinds of data to collect, when to let go, and when to move on. Most importantly, the third edition of *Basics* offers suggestions on how to capture the complexity in life and the variety of different ways persons respond to events in their lives through ongoing forms of inter/action and emotion. Keeping with and emphasizing what was so dear to Anselm Strauss, the third edition stresses the importance of putting process together with structure. It places action/interaction/emotional responses to events in the center stage and locates them within the larger historical, social, economic, political, etc. context in which events occur. And for those who want to develop theory, the book has a chapter on integration though it does not discourage persons whose interest is in doing thick rich description or case analysis from using some of the research techniques suggested in the book. Most of all, the methodology presented in the third edition of *Basics* emphasizes the need for researchers to take the time to think, observe, talk to diverse groups, compare, ask questions, follow the leads in the data, and write those memos.

Although grounded theorists today come from different perspectives and have their own approaches to analyzing data, I think certain threads run through all our methods, for example, doing comparative analysis and asking questions of the data, theoretical sampling, and writing memos. Concepts remain the foundation of research, along with the development of concepts in terms of their properties and dimensions. Other common threads are saturation and theoretical sampling, two concepts often misunderstood and misused by novices to qualitative research. For me, the importance of method is not whose approach one chooses but the "quality" of the research findings produced by any approach. Each of the methods here in this book has the potential to produce quality findings. In fact, looking at the list of evaluative criteria provided by Charmaz in her recent book *Constructing Grounded Theory* (2006), I find that any of them could be applied to the method described in the third edition of *Basics*. Findings have a way of speaking for themselves. Findings either resonate, offer new insights, explore phenomena in depth, add to a knowledge base, and make you stand up and listen or they don't. I personally don't see the purpose of all this hoopla about method. One could argue and discuss methods all day. In the end, it doesn't matter. People will choose the method that most speaks to them and they will use it in ways that make sense to them.

One last thought. I'm sure that if Anselm Strauss were alive today, he would say that his goal was to teach students how to think. He wanted to provide researchers with a methodology that would enable them to capture some of the complexity and variation in this world, qualities that add so much richness to life as we experience and live it as well as to our research findings. He wanted to give researchers the tools to produce findings that could be used to make the world a better place. He would be pleased to see the different methodological branches of grounded theory that have emerged from the second and third generation grounded theorists based upon the original work done by him and Barney Glaser (Glaser & Strauss, 1967). Though each of the contemporary and descendant methodologies is somewhat different, all have the capacity, if carried out properly, to do just what was intended—develop useful theory that is grounded in data.

References

Blumer, H. (1969). *Symbolic interactionism*. Englewood Cliffs, NJ: Prentice Hall.

Charmaz, K. (2006). *Constructing grounded theory*. Thousand Oaks, CA: Sage.

Clarke, A. E. (2005). *Situational analysis*. Thousand Oaks, CA: Sage.

Corbin, J. & Strauss, A. (2008). *Basics of qualitative research*, 3rd ed.. Thousand Oaks, CA: Sage.

Denzin, N. K. (1994). The art and politics of interpretation. In N. K. Denzin & Y. S. Lincoln (Eds.), *The Sage handbook of qualitative research* (pp. 500–515). Thousand Oaks, CA: Sage.

Denzin, N. K. (1998). The art and politics of interpretation. In N. K. Denzin & Y. S. Lincoln (Eds.), *Collecting and interpreting qualitative materials* (pp. 313–371). Thousand Oaks, CA: Sage.

Glaser, B. & Strauss, A. L. (1967). *The discovery of grounded theory*. Chicago: Aldine.

Hamberg, K. & Johansson E. (1999). Practitioner, researcher, and gender conflict in a qualitative study. *Qualitative Health Research*, 9(4), 455–467.

Hughes, E. C. (1971). *The sociological eye: Selected papers*. Chicago: Aldine-Atherton.

Olesen, V. (1998). Feminism and models of qualitative research. In N. K. Denzin & Y. S. Lincoln (Eds.), *The landscape of qualitative research theories and issues* (pp. 300–332). Thousand Oaks, CA: Sage.

Park, R. E. (1967). *On social control and collective behavior* (R. H. Turner, Ed.). Chicago: University of Chicago Press.

Schwandt, T. A. (1998). Constructivist, interpretivist approaches to human inquiry. In N. K. Denzin & Y. S. Lincoln (Eds.), *The landscape of qualitative research theories and issues* (pp. 221–259). Thousand Oaks, CA: Sage.

Strauss, A. L. & Corbin J. (1990). *Basics of qualitative research*. Thousand Oaks, CA: Sage.

Strauss, A. L. & Corbin J. (1998). *Basics of qualitative research*, 2nd ed. Thousand Oaks, CA: Sage.

Thomas, W. I. (1996). *On social control and collective behavior* (M. Janowitz, Ed.). Chicago: University of Chicago Press.

Dialogue: On "Cleaning" Transcripts

Q: I have heard a lot about cleaning the transcripts. My question is, does this cleaning decrease the richness of your data because you lose the tone from your answer?

Barbara: I don't have a lot to say about this but I think there is something lost in that I've also started to use tapes of interviews as well as transcripts. I think listening to the tapes adds a lot, adds another dimension. It adds some richness to the analysis.

Kathy: I agree I listen to tapes over and over and again. I've been criticized for the rationality of the [interview] accounts in my book and the person saying, not that I doctored the statements, so what was going on? What I concluded was that both rationality and emotionality were there. I encouraged Annika Lilrank, who is in Finland, to pursue the difference between the rationality of the story and emotion of the interview. The emotion that comes out during the talks is lost in the transcribed interview accounts but that emotion is nonetheless there, and I think that's really something to take note of.

Julie: I try not to. I think that you lose something if you do.

4. Glaserian Grounded Theory

Phyllis Noerager Stern

When during my doctoral studies at the University of California San Francisco (UCSF), I enrolled in the series of seminars named "The Discovery of Social Reality," first taught by Anselm Strauss, but after a couple of sessions by Barney Glaser, I felt like I had entered a social reality that had little to do with me. Sociology students made up most of the class and they spoke a language with which I was unfamiliar. I struggled until I finally made some sense of this strange jargon. My epiphany came after graduation, when I realized that one of my career tasks was to interpret the sociological jargon of Glaser and Strauss (1967), and Glaser (1978) into classical English.

Wait, that's a little too pat; in actuality, Covan and I wrote a grant application that never got funded, but the reviewers liked the method section. Salvaging that part of the proposal, Covan (then Maxwell) pub-lished it in a sociological journal (Max-well & Maxwell, 1980), and I rewrote that part of the proposal in the plainest English I could manage and submitted the manuscript to one of the leading nursing journals, *Image* (now called *The Journal of Nursing Scholarship*). The beauty of this journal is that it is member subscribed for a large international scholarly society and therefore widely read.

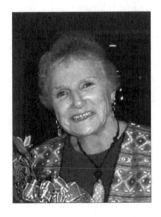

My timing was impeccable, but I didn't know that when I submitted the work. Holly

Wilson published the first grounded theory article in a nursing journal in 1977. It was a major breakthrough, but I thought her writing was still a bit too jargony. The *idea* of grounded theory swept through the nursing academic world as the method that could finally tell the world what it is that we do. The trouble was that nobody understood how to do it unless they had studied with Glaser and Strauss. (If you've read—or tried to read—*Discovery* you know what I mean.) Again, by the luck of the draw, just weeks after I had sent off the manuscript, the editor of *Image* called to say that another author had withdrawn her article. The editor asked if I could make a couple of changes so that *Image* could publish mine in the next issue (Stern, 1980). Talk about your heart-pounding moment! I didn't know if anybody would ever read it, but as a junior faculty member, I was most interested in putting another notch in my résumé belt. I've always tried to do good work, work that matters. But I had no idea that article would matter so much—scholars from all over North America came to me at scientific meetings to tell me they finally understood grounded theory. It also happened in New Zealand where I got to meet Pacific Rim scholars (Fourth International Congress on Women's Health Issues, 1990). For most of the 1980s, the article was required reading for nursing graduate students throughout the world. It was my interpretation of Glaserian grounded theory.

In this chapter, I will interpret the areas of Glaserian grounded theory for which Glaser gets attacked and then tell you a bit about *Sternian* grounded theory. Get it?—Stern, Sternian. Let's start with data and their worrisome accuracy. Charmaz (2006, p. 18) cites Dey's (1999) claim that Glaser and Strauss advocate "smash and grab" techniques when collecting data. To me, data collection needs to be guided by what the study is about. For example, Strauss was interested in how organizations work and the symbolic interaction between the players. Strauss relied on observation at the scene, making tape recorded notes after he left. For a more intimate and obviously emotional study, such as integration in stepfather families in which I did in-depth, sensitive interviews, close attention to body language was in order (Stern, 1981, 1982). Glaser's study of the subcontractor and the patsy was generated by personal experience and six months of detailed field notes (Glaser, 1976). I think we all agree with the truism: *Everything is data.* Glaser (2007) insists that grounded theory is a *method* that can be used with any kind of data. Currently, he and Holton are working on a book describing how one can apply grounded theory techniques to statistical data. Is he circling back to his work with descriptive statistics? We'll have to wait until the book comes out for the answer to that.

Notwithstanding possible boos from an audience, I confess that from my point of view, data accuracy is highly overrated. A grounded theory study is a theory generated from conglomerate data, interviews, observations, literature, or even statistics, so what difference does it make if Mary said, "I don't think I can go on," or "I just can't go on." The essence is there—*Going on* might be the substantive code. Let me explain further. Last year I worked with a Thai doctoral student, Pennapa Dangdomyouth (known to her friends as Nid), whose mastery of English was limited. A psych nurse, she wanted to know how Thai family caregivers manage their relatives with schizophrenia at home. She did interviews and observations and follow-up phone calls with eighteen caregivers. Then she needed to translate her data into English so I could read them and we could talk about them.

As you may know, Asian languages have a totally different sentence structure from Western languages—there's no such thing as a direct translation. The field notes came out in pigeon English, and, although technically inaccurate, the substance of the interviews remained. I think you'll agree that when a woman said, "I watch him with corner eye," it may not hold up as grammatically correct, but you get what she means. After examining all the data, and knowing what we know about the behavior of individuals suffering with schizophrenia, and realizing that Thai culture had earned its way into the theory, we were able to come up with the core category, which became the subject of the article: "Tactful Monitoring: How Thai Caregivers Manage Their Relative with Schizophrenia at Home" (Dangdomyouth et al., 2008). Nid earned her PhD in July 2007.

Nurses, in particular, find the concept of worrisome accuracy troubling. No surprise; in our work, we *have* to be accurate. Covan thinks the more competent the practitioner, the less likely it is that a researcher can understand the basic concepts of grounded theory; how it is that you have to break the rules to get the job done (Covan, personal communication, September 11, 2007). I see doing grounded theory as a creative process— if you really want to know what's going on, you have to feel it; you have to be affected by it; you have to let it move you. Objectivity has *no place* in qualitative research. When I did my stepfather study back in the 1970s, tape recorders were large cumbersome things. No way was I going to lug one of those around to people's homes. Besides, I thought the recording might be off putting to the people I talked with. I wrote field notes instead; I got pretty good at writing while maintaining eye contact. Then I typed up the interview as soon as possible. Were the data inaccurate? Possibly, but as I typed up the notes, I could hear their voices, see their nonverbal movements, see how their living room or their kitchen was arranged. If I heard distress, I felt distressed for days.

If I didn't record each word exactly, did it damage the final outcome of the study? I truly believe it did not. Why? Because a grounded theory is a theoretical interpretation of a conglomerate of data rather than a case report of a series of incidents. I was the instrument, and my worldview went into the mix. But I didn't find what I expected to before beginning the study because I *had to respect the data*. In the study I'm working on with Covan about cadet nurses during World War II,[1] we used video tape, not remembering my ideas about recording being off putting—we were going to make a documentary until we realized we didn't know how. The nurses were my classmates in training in the 1940s. My plan was to do the interviews myself, but most of the former cadets lived in a variety of California sites. California is a big state, and after driving half a day to an interview, I realized I hadn't the stamina to finish the job. Two Master's students conducted about half of the interviews using a camcorder with a tripod and a script.

With a couple of exceptions, at the end of the interview the former cadets exhaled and said, "That wasn't as bad as I expected." Those data were accurate but stiff, which belied their accuracy. Get it? For instance, Suzy Sanders, one of the most effusive and jolly of the group, came across as up-tight and shy; that wasn't the real Suzy, so the data weren't real. I also ended up with too much data and insufficiently directed interviews that didn't follow the emerging theory. Not that we're throwing anything away, mind you; with more examination of the data, we have discovered a core category. How do cadet nurses at a San Francisco training school during World War II remember the experience? *It was fun.* The fun was the pleasures of the big city with lots of available military service men, school dances, and the camaraderie of the nurses' dorm. We were also doing our patriotic duty.

Over the past ten years especially, I have heard the language of grounded theory criticized as being positivistic. Well, yeah, Glaser and Strauss were writing to that audience—trying to help positivistic sociologists understand that there was another legitimate way to approach data.

Glaser and Strauss were interpreting grounded theory for the positivists. Barney reasons that the language of grounded theory needs to have consistency over time. To me, it's no big deal. Although I'm told that language guides thought, and all of that, to me, the big deal is putting forth work that can be easily understood by as many readers as possible. Some people object to the use of the term "emergence" as the way one finally discovers theory from data. Well, the theory certainly doesn't rise up off the page as the term implies, but after weeks or months of painstaking analysis when you finally get it, it seems like a second coming. And I rather like the phrase, "trust in emergence," which is a warning to new and seasoned researchers alike to avoid imposing preexisting frameworks on the data.

Glaser is also criticized for running a vanity press—publishing his works through his own company, Sociology Press. I asked him if the press published anything besides his work. I think he was a little irked when he wrote:

Yes, in the many readers other people's stuff abounds including yours. We have 6 readers, organizational careers, examples of GT [grounded theory], GT 84-94, BSP [basic social process] dissertations, more grounded theory methodology, the GT seminar reader; thus 100's of other people's work. (electronic communication, July 5, 2007)

Barney's take on it is that he's doing the authors in his readers a favor by publishing their work; seriously, he's enormously proud of his protégés' work and he *remembers* what they found. I confess I feel flattered when an article of mine, published elsewhere, is included. As well, he thinks examples of grounded theories should be gathered together for a handy reference guide. In the introduction to his latest reader (Glaser & Holton, 2007), he quotes a passage he wrote in 1993:

It became obvious to me that what was needed by the myriad GT readers, researchers, and users throughout the world was a book of examples of GT papers and chapters. Researchers need models for how the various facets of GT look when brought together into an integrated piece. (p. ix)

At the School of Nursing at UCSF, the grounded theory dissertation model most students used was Holly Wilson's 1975 study of Soteria House, an alternative treatment facility for the mentally ill. I still have the one I copied (Holly, a nurse, earned her terminal degree in educational psychology at Berkeley). The authors of these grounded theory readers don't share in the profits of Glaser's publications, but there are other rewards in academia, and having articles reprinted in collections helps attain them. Among the twenty-three publications offered by Sociology Press are otherwise out-of-print books by other writers. Aware of Glaser's career, when the fourth publisher in the 2006–2007 period asked me for a piece on grounded theory (celebrating forty years of grounded theory was a heads-up for publishers), I was moved to ask, "What's in it for me?" The publisher responded, "The usual academic rewards" (electronic communication with Mitchell Allen, November 15, 2006). But I've been a full professor since 1980 and I have all the awards I'm likely to get. Shouldn't we get advances or something?

Glaser, in his writing seems to be evolving, in that he emphasizes a variety of aspects of doing grounded theory; although he takes pains to deny that he has changed anything! Process, he insists in his 2005 book, is but one theoretical code out of an infinite number. He cites his 1978 book to prove the consistency of his position. In the 2005 book, he lists a number of codes that have been used to good effect but warns against developing "pet" codes, where one discovers a theoretical code and likes it so well that one applies it to all subsequent data. He writes that Strauss saw everything as pacing, but only freed himself of his pet code when he discovered the conditional matrix. The problem with a pet code is that it imposes a framework on the data, rather than allowing the theory to emerge. If a theoretical code has sufficient *grab*, he tells us, it can be the framework of whole departments and it can make careers; for example, some authors "sponsor" constructionist interpretation of symbolic interaction. Further, Glaser (2005) names *names*:

> For example, Strauss pushes process and conditional matrix. R. K. Merton always pushed role status, Berry Gibson pushes autopoiesis, and Granovetter pushes networks. And Lincoln and Guba push mutual shaping as a replacement of causal theory. Students, as apprentices, working under these people or their students are caught by the grab for a long time, if not forever. (p. 107)

Benoliel (2001) wrote that the influence of phenomenology on grounded theory methods has enhanced their usefulness. For my part, I always had the impression that we constructed grounded theory—we built it. Sorting memos by hand, we built piles of thoughts about data that became the grounded theory. And symbolic interactionism may be a theoretical code, but one ignores it at one's peril, especially when one studies situations important to my profession, nursing. But it may not be the most important thing that's going on. It may be part of the mixture that's derived from the data.

I edited a peer-reviewed journal, *Health Care for Women International*, for twenty years. I also review for a number of other journals. As a consequence, I read many grounded theory manuscripts. The first thing I do is check the reference list to see if my name is there. Then I look for Glaser and/or Glaser and Strauss, or Clarke or Charmez or Wuest—someone I know to be solid. If the authors failed to cite these authorities, I know I'm in for a rough read. Usually. Where authors tend to mess up is in halting their constant comparison before they develop a theory. In a paper I read recently, the authors came up with three categories. It was pretty easy for me, the grayback, to see how the categories were interconnected, so I could give the authors some helpful feedback. Back to my original warning: Variations on grounded theory are all well and good, but it is important to understand the original concepts; the most vital of these may be constant comparison until the researcher finds a theoretical code that has fit and grab.

Is a given grounded theory the only answer to a research question? Absolutely not. A grounded theorist makes choices like any other researcher. When I did the stepfamily study, I followed the trail of disciplining children, which later broadened to include childrearing. I could have chosen the financial problems, a factor in all marriages. But I made a choice. After I did a study with Filipino immigrants (Stern, 1981), I reexamined my stepfamily data and discovered a condition I called "individual family culture" (Stern 1982). The mother has her family cultural values, as does the stepfather, and the child has the values of mother, biological father, and divorced mother living; all have clear and persistent beliefs about right and wrong. When these individuals come together, culture shock ensues and they're ripe for a session with TV psychologist Dr. Phil. In the study of survivors of home fires (Stern & Kerry, 1996), we found that there was often no *comforting* ritual for these victims. At one time I thought there was *no* ritual, but Jan Morse pointed out that there's no such thing as no ritual (personal communication, 1984). I could have studied first responders, or the support of the church, but I made a choice. Someone else might find something different. That's why grounded theory can never be replicated—the population is different, the researcher is different, the time is different. This is a postmodern world, and now that I know what the term means, I can become fluent in the lingo.

So why are Glaser's protégés so loyal? Because he's so *there*. If you think you're stumbling, you can call him or e-mail him and get his advice. (Strauss was like that as well.) Barney's the kind of a genius who talks like a genius—too intellectual for us regular people to understand. I've done workshops with him where I acted as interpreter to help a bewildered audience make sense of what he was saying. But he does OK by himself. His main occupation, other than writing books, is conducting trouble-shooting workshops mainly for PhD students. In his latest reader, he published twenty-four papers from the workshops. To him, grounded theory is a universal method that works for any professional. I agree.

Glaser and Strauss introduced the concept of formal grounded theory in the *Discovery* book. Glaser revisited the idea in 2007 (Glaser, 2007). I haven't read any rebuttal to this book, but maybe it hasn't been out long enough for that. The advantage of a formal grounded theory is that it is more generalizable. Status passage, for example, *could* pertain to the situations along the passage from boy to man. No one incident, the bar mitzvah say, which for Jewish boys is an important ceremony declaring their manhood, really creates a man from a thirteen-year-old boy. There are many benchmarks ahead before this adolescent takes on the mantle of grown man, with all its duties and responsibilities.

Glaser tells us that to develop a formal theory from a substantive theory, the researcher needs to follow the core category rather than beginning with a research question, but he warns that the search need not exceed the researcher's resources or energy. From time to time, I have thought about trying to develop formal theory from a substantive theory, but while holding a full-time job, it just seemed too arduous a task—in truth, I abhor searching the literature. But life is a continuing learning process, and in these, my declining years, I have learned how to use the computer to search the literature for me. Suddenly, formal theory seems doable. But I still have questions. On Sunday, September 9, 2007, Barney and I had this e-mail exchange:

Hi Barn,

There's this push among qualitative researchers to publish qualitative synthesis to rival quantitative meta analysis. Now, I get that to develop formal theory you follow the core variable, but my take is that if I were to gather data for a formal theory, I would search the literature that added to the core category regardless of the method. Do you agree?

Phyllis

Phyllis, thanks for the memo. I am in the midst of writing the chapter on quantitative vs./and/or qualitative GT. Yes, search the literature for items on the core variable, BUT be sure to look at the type and cogency of the method behind it as part of conceptual comparison, NOT comparative description.

Barn

I'm not sure I understand this message, but I think he's advising me to keep the comparison on the conceptual level rather than describing the substantive findings. He does tell us that a formal theory will have fewer examples to explain how the formal theory is derived then does a substantive theory. He tells us that formal theory development takes a seasoned grounded theorist—it would be too much at the dissertation level: "Beginners have enough trouble doing SGT [substantive grounded theory]" (Glaser 2007, p. 83).

Has grounded theory evolved? Yes and no. If the word had been around at the time, I think, to put it in a book title, Glaser and Strauss would have called the method "constructionist," but it took Kathy Charmaz to do so (Charmaz, 2006). Glaser and Strauss taught us that everything is data, including the worldview of the researcher, although they put it in different terms. Adele Clarke adds history to her analysis; how about this for a book title: *Situational Analysis: Grounded Theory after the Postmodern Turn* (Clarke, 2005). Barbara Bowers, who worked with Lenny Schatzman, uses dimensional analysis (Pandhi, Bowers, & Chen, in press). Judy Wuest (2001) uses a feminist perspective as a theoretical code and has managed to impact policy change as a consequence. Covan's work with the elderly during hurricane rescue has changed the way first responders, well, respond (Covan et al., 2001; Rosenkoetter et al., 2007). All of these researchers stick to the basic principals of the method.

Finally, how have I evolved as interpreter of the method? In every paper I write, I think I add more clarity to how you do this stuff. I learn from my students what to emphasize, what to leave out, and hopefully I leave them lovin' it. When I'm 100, maybe I'll get it right.

Note

1. The Cadet Nurse Corps was a highly successful U.S. government–funded program aimed at recruiting student nurses during World War II to alleviate a severe nursing shortage in civilian hospitals. Upon graduation, cadet nurses were pledged to serve in military forces or public health venues.

References

Benoliel, J. Q. (2001). Expanding knowledge about women through grounded theory: Introduction to the collection. *Health Care for Women International*, 22, 1–3.

Charmaz, K. (2006). *Constructing grounded theory*. Thousand Oaks, CA: Sage.

Clarke, A. E. (2005). *Situational analysis: Grounded theory after the postmodern turn*. Thousand Oaks, CA: Sage.

Covan, E. K., Rosenkoetter, M. M., Richards, B., & Lane, A. (2001). The impact of Hurricane Floyd on the elderly residing in four southeastern North Carolina counties. In J. R. Maiolo, J. C. Whitehead, M. McGee, L. King, J. Johnson, & Harold Stone (Eds.), *Facing our future: Hurricane Floyd and the recovery in the coastal plain* (pp. 213–233). Wilmington, NC: Coastal Carolina Press.

Dangdomyouth, P., Stern, P. N., Oumtanee, A., & Yunibhand, J. (2008). Tactful monitoring: How Thai caregivers manage their relative with schizophrenia at home. *Issues in Mental Nursing*, 29, 37–50.

Dey, I. (1999). *Grounding grounded theory*. San Diego: Academic Press.

Fourth International Congress on Women's Health Issues (1990). Palmerston North, New Zealand, November 15–18.

Glaser, B. G. (1964). *Organizational scientists: Their professional careers*. New York: Bobbs Merrill

Glaser, B. G. (1972/76). *Experts versus laymen: A study of the patsy and the subcontractor*. Mill Valley: Sociology Press.

Glaser, B. G. (1978). *Theoretical sensitivity*. Mill Valley, CA: Sociology Press

Glaser, B. G. (1993). *Examples of grounded theory: A reader*. Mill Valley, CA: Sociology Press.

Glaser, B. G. (2005). *The grounded theory perspective III: Theoretical coding*. Mill Valley, CA: Sociology Press.

Glaser, B. G. (2007). *Doing formal grounded theory: A proposal*. Mill Valley, CA: Sociology Press.

Glaser, B. G. & Holton, J. A. (2007). *The grounded theory seminar reader*. Mill Valley, CA: Sociology Press.

Glaser, B. G. & Strauss, A. L. (1967). *The discovery of grounded theory*. Chicago: Aldine.

Maxwell. E. K., & Maxwell, R. J. (1980). Search and research in ethnology: Continuous comparative analysis. *Behavior Science Research*, 15, 219–243.

Pandhi, N., Bowers, B., Chen, F. (In press) A comfortable relationship: A patient derived dimension of ongoing care. *Family Medicine*.

Rosenkoetter, M. M., Covan, E. K., Cobb, B. K., Bunting, S., & Weinrich, M. (2007). Perceptions of older adults regarding evacuation in the event of a natural disaster. *Public Health Nursing*, 24(2), 160–168.

Stern, P. N. (1980). Grounded theory methodology: Its uses and processes. *Image: The Journal of Nursing Scholarship*, 12, 20–23.

Stern, P. N. (1981). Solving problems of cross-cultural health teaching: The Filipino childbearing family. *Image*, 13, 47–50.

Stern, P. N. (1982). Conflicting family culture: An impediment to integration in stepfather families. *Journal of Psychosocial Nursing*, 20, 27–33.

Stern, P. N. & Kerry, J. (1996). Restructuring life after home loss by fire. *Image: The Journal of Nursing Scholarship*, 28, 9–14.

Wilson, H. S. (1977). Limited intrusion: Social control of outsiders in a healing community. *Nursing Research*, 26, 105–111.

Wuest, J. (2001). Precarious ordering: Towards a formal theory of women's caring. *Health Care for Women International*, 22, 167–193.

Example: Restructuring Life after Home Loss by Fire

Phyllis Noerager Stern and June Kerry

Introduction

Victims of home fires generally receive a "ritual-support connection" from their social network. A study of 113 people from eight countries shows social ritual, not need, leads the support for home fire victims. Connected support fills the victims' short-term needs and is prevalent in rural settings. Unconnected support to victims is the most common and is often misdirected or insulting. People restructure their lives after a fire by limiting their display of grief and developing new ways to prevent fires.

When fire destroys a home, victims endure the disorientation, feelings of helplessness, sadness, and depletion that are engendered by privation and the problem of restructuring their lives. The research questions in this grounded theory study were: How do victims process losing their homes to fire? How does social ritual connect with their needs? We found that, despite the seriousness of the problems victims face, social ritual guides support. In many instances, this ritual dictates support that is short term and only loosely related to the actual needs of victims. In other words, the support that victims receive is determined by social ritual rather than need. We have named this "ritual-support connection," the dimensions of which are (1) connected support, (2) unconnected support, and (3) disconnected support. In a noncomforting social framework, victims must integrate the salient life event of home loss by fire, through a process we have named "restructuring life." Two dimensions of restructuring are limiting grief displays and developing new rituals. New rituals include benchmarking, taking precautions, and becoming expert.

Material possessions hold symbolic meaning for us. Acquisitions, in addition to their market value, call up memories of when and where they were purchased, who was involved, and who found the possessions of worth. We value things we own for their beauty, their connection to ancestors, or because they are necessary to our survival. When our possessions are reduced to rubble by flames, parts of our lives are destroyed as well.

Home fires differ from other disasters in that, generally, fire strikes one household at a time. The support of ongoing social services and the shared experience of disaster victims are missing in most home fires. The exception is massive disasters such as the San Francisco fire of 1906, or the Oakland fire of 1991, where the attention of an entire community focused on the event and its survivors. In contrast, for individual home fires, many victims have nowhere to turn for comfort.

Significance

As Northrup (1989) reports, in Canada (the country in which the major data collection for this study took place), there were 67,884 fires in 1987, in which 555 individuals lost their lives. Property damage amounted to over $973 million in Canadian currency. The Nova Scotia fire Marshall reported in 1984 that overall, residential fires accounted for 53% of the total number of reported fires in that province and more than 90% of fatal fires. "Between April 1, 1987, and March 31, 1988 [Labor Minister Terry Donahoe] said, more than 2,300 fires occurred in Nova Scotia [a province with a population equal to San Francisco], killing 36 people and causing almost $20 million in damage" (National Fire Investigation, 1988, p. 8). In more recent reports, the National Fire Prevention Association Survey lists 459,000 home fires in the United States in 1992, which caused 3,705 deaths and 21,100 injuries. Although loss of homes from fires is relatively commonplace, ritual and social support studies concerning recovery have not yet been reported. Our purpose was to discover the experiences of home loss by fire. We hoped to identify areas for appropriate intervention by mental health, community health, and burn-unit nurses.

Grounded Theory Methodology

Grounded theory methodology, developed by Glaser and Strauss (1967) has been used extensively to address questions of interest to researchers. An investigator's purpose in using grounded theory is to develop a theory, grounded in data gathered during a given study, rather than testing theory developed by other scientists (Glaser, 1978, 1992, 1993, 1994; Glaser & Strauss, 1967; Stern, 1980, 1985, 1991, 1994; Stem, Allen, & Moxley, 1982; Strauss, 1987). As Glaser (1992) puts it, a researcher attempts to discover the chief problem in a given situation, from the perspective of the participants, and how participants process the problem.

Every research method has its own jargon. For example in quantitative research, terms such as multiple regression, factor analysis, ANOVA, t-tests, and degrees of freedom are common, and results are reported using measures of significance. Qualitative methods also have their own special jargon; this is one way readers distinguishes one method from another (Baker, Wuest, & Stern, 1992). For example, phenomenologists speak of, "the lived experience" of participants and "bracket data," whereas anthropologists use techniques of "participant observation" and rely on "chief informants" to find particular truths (Stern, 1994).

In the language of grounded theory, data are manipulated by "constant comparison" to develop "hypotheses" (hunches). Findings are reported in terms of explanations about what the researcher thinks is a workable hypothesis. The hypothesis, usually called a "core variable" or "central process," is made up of a number of "social psychological processes" (processes wherein the psychological outlook of a person is affected by the response of society, seen through "symbolic act") and "social structural processes" (processes governed by the structure or rules of society). These processes occur within a given "context" or scene. A grounded theory research report is a description of how the processes make up the discovered theory and often includes a comparison of how this theory and existing theory adds to our knowledge.

Fire Victims

In our study of home fire victims, data were collected between 1987 and

1992. Our research originated with a single case study of a victim who suffered painful sociopsychological sequelae following home loss by fire. It became clear to us that this was a fruitful area for study. Following institutional ethical approval, we adhered to the principle of grounded theory, which posits that our sample selection be dictated by the developing hypothesis. In grounded theory, no hard and fast rules exist about sample inclusion or exclusion; the design of grounded theory is one of exploration, not a mapped course. In other words, no map exists and the researcher is the map maker. In our sample selection, we required only that victims had lost their dwellings to fire, or that damage had been so extensive that they had been forced to vacate the premises, and that participants spoke either English or French. A precise description of a sample in terms of numbers of a certain age, race, income, and the like is ordinarily excluded from a grounded theory report (Stern, 1991).

Our first participants were referrals from colleagues. We talked with anyone we could find who had experienced a home fire. As we analyzed the first interviews, we began to form hypotheses. To be true to the method, we selected participants on the basis of their ability to help us solve the puzzle of what surviving a fire symbolized for them. That is, we used a purposive sample: participants who suited our purpose of solving the mystery. For example, as we formed hypotheses about recent fire victims, we looked for survivors whose personal disaster occurred earlier in their lives. When we were told, "Folks in the country help out each other," we concentrated for a time on victims whose fire occurred in rural settings. As the ritual-support connection category became apparent, we investigated home loss by fire in other cultures, talking with individuals of diverse cultures whenever the opportunity arose.

Connection sites were mainly the southeastern Canadian provinces of Nova Scotia (n = thirty), New Brunswick (n = thirty-five) and Prince Edward Island (n = four). Both English- and French-speaking Canadians participated. Additional data were collected from victims in California (n = eight), Texas (n = four), Oregon (n = two), New York (n = three), and Detroit (n = one). Data about ritual were also collected during short interviews in Denmark (n = eight), Sweden (n = seven), Australia (n = three), Korea (n = four), China (n = two), New Zealand (n = three), and Fiji (n = one). Many of the victims in Canada and the United States complained about their interactions with insurance representatives and public service employees. Therefore, we asked some representatives from these service sectors who had worked with home fire victims to participate in the study.

Using traditional techniques of grounded theory (Glaser, 1992), data were examined, coded for substance, categorized, expanded, reduced, and subjected to coding in overlapping processes, thus allowing the central activity of restructuring life to emerge. We found that the victims' difficulty in recovering from home fires was exacerbated because, generally, no comforting social ritual supported them in working through their difficulty. A typical comment leading to this conclusion was, "It's like people want to do something, but they don't know what to do."

Once developed, the analysis was presented to selected fire victims in the United States and Canada who had been particularly informative ($n =$ twenty) for checks on accuracy and fit with their perceptions of the problem of restructuring their lives after a home fire and how they processed it. Then we concentrated on the importance of ritual, that is, on prescribed symbolic behavior to the recovery process in home fire because the absence of comforting ritual seemed to be an aspect of the study that would be amenable to nursing intervention.

Impact of the Disaster

In describing the effect of home fires, informants spoke of the loss as being akin to losing a family member to death, because often the articles burned had been given to them by a deceased relative. Victims spoke of feeling physically ill at the sight of their burned possessions.

Wandering Aimlessly

Victims went through a period of being disoriented and disorganized; some even hallucinated. Purposive action at this time was almost impossible. Kerry (1991) called this "wandering," and Northrup (1989) named it "stepping in and out of reality." In his study of the fire in Coconut Grove California, Lindemann (1944/1965) described survivors' grief reactions as anger, loss of energy, and guilt. In the present study, the strongest memory that victims had was of disorientation because of the loss of the place where grief is usually expressed—their home. In spite of their helplessness, victims were forced to take on the task of restoration and restructuring.

Restructuring Life

Losing the fabric of their lives—the very structure in which they retreated to feel safe—victims told us they had to "start from scratch." Fire victims had to rebuild their lives along with their dwellings. For fire victims, the physical work of restoration seemed more difficult than mourning the death of a family member because the tools with which to do the restoring—records, books, even pencils and papers—had been destroyed. Victims, while working through the grief of loss, needed to find a place to sleep, something to sleep on, and clothes to wear. Shopping became an arduous task. Uninsured victims suffered terrible financial problems—sometimes never recouping the losses. When a victim was insured, endless lists of home contents needed to be compiled—often from memory. Furthermore, victims needed to continue to fulfill obligations of employment.

Dimensions of the Ritual-Support Connection

Anthropologists tell us that ritual in the lives of everyone, regardless of culture, is vital to well-being (Olien, 1978). Bright (1990) stated, "Ritual is prescribed symbolic behavior that defines and is defined by interactions among people, within the larger social context, for the purpose of addressing changing needs" (p. 24). Ritual importance is learned through watching, by being actively taught, by imitation, and by correction (Maxwell, 1993). There is little research on ritual in health care (Davis-Floyd, 1990; Jackson, 1984; Wolin & Bennett, 1984), and, although there are a number of instructive articles about ritual in nursing practice (Farrington, 1990; Huey, 1986; Huttmann, 1985; Walker, 1967, Welsh & Ford, 1989a, 1989b, 1989c), only two research-based articles were located (Schmahl, 1964; Wolf, 1988). The ritual friends and acquaintances follow with house fire victims is simple, short, and uncomforting, usually consisting of questions about injury and monetary loss. These friends and acquaintances expressed sympathy, but little further support. Victims are forced to process their loss in a climate of ritual-support disconnection, that is, with little comforting.

When we cross-tabulated the data on ritual and support, we found three dimensions of support, including informed support, no support (or neglect), and uninformed support such as insults; another dimension is time limits. As one victim told us, "Sometimes it seems like what people think they ought to do for you has no connection with what you need." Therefore, we named the dimensions of the ritual-support connection (1) connected, where support is connected to need; (2) unconnected, in which ritual fails to bring about comforting support; and (3) disconnected, where comforting ritual is withheld from victims thought to be unworthy of support. Although support may be absent, there is never a total absence of ritual for a given situation. The ritual may be to ignore the victim, an "it's-not-my-business," response. Therefore, in our cross-tabulation we had no data for a dimension of no support and no ritual.

Connected Support

Generally, we found rituals following fires in rural settings to be comforting and connected to need. Morse (1992) defines the concept of comforting:

> The outcome of comforting [i.e., feeling comfortable] was described as a change in mood, as a "warm feeling of relief," "feeling confident," feeling "in touch with one's self," [sic] and "at ease. ..." The comforting response of the comforter, the "reaching out" to the other, is reflexive and focused on the sufferer. (p. 95)

In rural settings, where social services are sparse, neighbors fill the breach by "looking out for each other—you'd die out here if you didn't." People who dwell in rural areas know they must depend on one another for survival. Country neighbors and friends often provide victims with a place to live, food, and clothing. Sometimes they rebuilt victims' homes. These are properties of ritual-support connection. When we described the devastation of loss suffered by fire victims to a man from a rural area in the province of Prince Edward Island, he explained how country ritual is connected to need: "Why we'd have those folks fixed up in no time. By nightfall, they'd have a place to sleep, clothes to wear, and the neighbors would bring them food for a couple of weeks. And we'd keep watching out for them too. Island folks know what to do."

We found evidence of comforting ritual (connected to need) for fire victims in the rural areas of North America, China, Denmark, Sweden, Australia, and New Zealand. We were told that in Germany, there is a saying that, "Having a fire is like moving three times," which denotes the enormity of the loss. In Korea, participants said that victims are told they will come into great wealth. When asked if neighbors helped victims attain wealth, the response was, "No, but at least the loss is acknowledged."

We found supportive ritual was more likely forthcoming when victims suffered a burn injury or a family member died. For death and injury, we have comforting rituals—hence victims and support people "knew what they were supposed to do, so they could help."

Unconnected Support

Overwhelmingly, our data indicate a variable we call unconnected ritual-support, that is, common ritual that has little or no connection to the actual needs of victims. Where support for victims was offered, it was generally of short duration, misdirected, or insulting. The most neglected victims had nowhere to turn for support and had few social connections generally. When disaster struck, they were stranded. Categories of unconnected support identified include unintended insults, neglect, misdirected support, withheld permission to grieve, and time dimensions.

Unintended Insult. Members of a victim's social network sometimes inflicted unintended insults. These included comments such as, "You're really lucky to be able to buy all new things," and "Oh, what fun to do all that shopping." Although the remark, "You're so lucky no one was hurt" was accepted as truth, the implication to the victim was, "so you have nothing to complain about." A home fire often carries a stigmatizing component, suggesting victim carelessness. Victims were commonly asked if they had left on an iron, clothes dryer, or hair dryer. An arson victim was asked, "What did you do [to cause this]?"

Neglect. Victims often suffered neglect described by one woman this way: "They say, 'Oh how sad, how awful,' and they just go on with their lives ... they don't really know it is just sort of like a death."

A young girl's friends at school apparently had no models of appropriate behavior following a home loss, so they ignored the event. The girl said: "I think they were too scared. Like, they might say something wrong that I wouldn't like ... or they thought that I wouldn't want to talk about it." Although these were ten year olds, their reaction to loss was much the same as the reports of adults' behavior.

The most neglected victims described themselves as having "nowhere-to-turn." These victims tended to be alike geographically and in having extremely weak social networks. In the study population, these neglected victims were city dwellers. One woman said, "You know how it is in the city, you don't want to know your neighbors that well." Unlike victims who had a close social network that afforded connected support, these victims had few social contacts in general. The stereotypical victim who had nowhere to turn was an older woman who had moved to smaller quarters in the city after the death of a spouse. A number of single mothers who were estranged from their family of origin fell into this category as well. For people in this category who were insured, the main support person was often the insurance adjustor—adjustors were there, offering to inventory the lost possessions, and usually granting financial assistance. They were just a call away. But their loyalty was to their company. The adjustor was engaged in a process that Hutchinson (1983) called covering: covering all the bases; making sure everything was done properly; offering compensation only after a complete list of contents was made out by the victim, and finally, covering the material needs of the insured. One adjustor put it this way: "I guess we have to initially go into all of the things that we also do when we prepare a case or conduct an investigation ... in the back of your mind, it's under the assumption that it may go to trial."

Misdirected support. People who did want to help had learned no comforting ritual to guide them. One victim who had suffered severe financial loss stated:

A lot of people wanted to do something but of course didn't know what to do. ... Actually, this is really hard to tell people, but money would help. But what happened was ... they'd come by and drop off things they were going to send to the Goodwill, basically junk. ... They were trying to help but it made it worse. It made you feel like you were living on the street.

Withheld permission to grieve. Victims were allowed to grieve openly when there was death or injury. However, grief over the loss of material things was disallowed. Victims were reminded of their good fortune at being alive and uninjured. One man said: "People tell you that you only lost 'things,' and they say it like it was trash, 'things!' They expect you to pull up your socks and get on with it. Maybe they were just things but those things helped me remember my life. ... They discount your grief."

For Fire Victims, the Loss of Possessions Is Trivialized

Time Dimensions

Even when grief was seen as legitimate, the connection of support to need generally fell short of the mark. For example, the social nexus of survivors seemed to consider a legitimate grieving period for death of a significant other as about a year and the appropriate grief time for burn injury was seen as somewhat less. Victims were told: "Get on with it," "Pull yourself together," and "It's best not to talk about it." Although connected support was offered in cases of death or injury, it was time limited and seen by most victims as insufficient, and therefore not connected to need.

Disconnected Support

Where comforting ritual does exist, but is withheld on the basis of social judgments, we find the third dimension of the ritual-support process—disconnected support. We found that support can be offered on the basis of perceived need, but the social worth of the recipient enters into the equation. A disconnected victim is seen by other members of society as unworthy of support, as if the victim were somehow to blame for the fire. For example, one participant told us that on Detroit television, although more reported fires cover loss suffered by black families, when fire victims are white, the story runs longer. This participant commented:

I guess since there are a lot of poor black people here, there's a general feeling that poor and careless go together—never mind that the landlord may be the one who doesn't tend to faulty electrical wiring. White people are better copy, because they get more sympathy. Ergo, white people are more careful, so Blacks deserve to get burned out.

A woman who lost a brother and a cousin in a fire and was severely burned herself said that the family received little support and she assumed it was because they lived in the wrong part of town. She said, "The part of town that we were living in … we are nothing compared to everybody else. When we have a fire, they blame us."

For victims without insurance, the Red Cross and Salvation Army were sources of short-term support providing clothing, food, and temporary shelter. For insured victims, these agencies were nonoptions—they never thought about it. No victims we interviewed sought support from their pastors, even though many were devoutly religious. Psychotherapy was chosen by a limited number of victims—all Americans in this sample.

Restructuring Life

Fire victims soon realized that if they were to survive—become survivors (Northrup, 1989)—they had to begin restructuring their lives. This comment was typical:

> It's just so hard to think that you have to start all over—that there's just nothing anymore. No walls, no guidelines, nothing. And nobody's going to do it for you. It's hard to know what to do first, but you just have to do it. I mean, how do you rebuild a whole life?

Furthermore, over time it became clear to victims that the rebuilding (restructuring) must take place within a society where the rules of conduct (social structural process) are governed by "ritual support connection"; that is, for victims who received connected support, the restructuring—though painful—was undertaken within a milieu of appropriate comforting measures. Those people who restructured their lives where there was unconnected or disconnected ritual-support received less or no comforting. Participants with stamina and relevant life experiences seemed able to regroup more quickly and with less lasting trauma.

All survivors agreed that restructuring is painful, but some were able to complete the task more easily than others. One man said, "You can't control what happens to you but you can control how you respond." His wife explained, "We've had a lot of adversity in our lives. I think that helps to make you strong." Their neighbor—also a victim—agreed" "Our life had just gone on like it was supposed to until this happened. We had a terrible time adjusting to the fact that we were wiped out."

The "remodeling" process that Scheela (1992) described in recovering incest offenders is similar to the restructuring that fire victims describe. The world of discovered incest offenders "falls apart," and offenders are faced with the prospect of rebuilding their lives. Although incest offenders may choose to remodel their lives, fire victims felt they had no choice.

Limiting the Display of Grief

Survivors longed for comforting understanding. However, in the social world in which they lived, extended expressions of grief and disorientation were usually discouraged. One woman explained:

> After a while, people's eyes start to glaze over and you know they're getting bored with your troubles. I felt pretty crazy but I've been around long enough to know that once you admit that you're losing it, people never forget it—you never live it down. No, it's just not socially correct to be nuts. By losing status among their peers and thus becoming more discomfited, survivors limited the display of their grief.

Developing New Rituals

When they found no comforting social rituals, fire survivors developed their own set of rituals to comfort themselves. Common rituals were benchmarking, taking precautions, and becoming expert.

Benchmarking

As part of their transcendence from victim to survivor, the fire became a marker for other life events. We were told by a survivor of the San Francisco fire of 1906 that individuals marked the rest of their lives by that disaster: Events were labeled as occurring "before" or "after" the fire. There is evidence that survivors of the 1991 Oakland fire will do the same. A victim whose house burned to the ground in that fire said, "It's been a year, so I guess I'll make it." All survivors in this study marked their progress in a similar way.

Taking Precautions

Many survivors became meticulous fire preventers. They developed rituals about unplugging appliances, checking the fire extinguisher, and closing fireplace screens. An arson victim said, "It wasn't even my fault but still I check everything. I don't know if I could do it [complete the recovery] again."

Becoming Expert

Some survivors began advising others in their social network about fire prevention. One survivor, who considered the fire company incompetent, started a movement to enhance fire fighters' efficiency in his city. He said, "I gave a talk to the Lion's Club on fire prevention. I figured something good should come out of all this." Survivors developed the ritual of becoming experts as a way of repairing damage to themselves.

Toward Developing New Social Rituals

A taxi driver from Fiji described a ritual that seemed to address the problem of the symbolic meaning of burned possessions. In rural Fiji, villagers rebuild the homes of fire victims. In addition, if a sacred object is lost, they make a duplicate: "It is not the same because the old one was maybe 1,000 years old. So we bless the new one and then it becomes 1,000 years old."

It is doubtful that a similar ritual could be developed in North America. We suggest that in its place, a ritual of support groups for fire victims needs to be developed. Support groups would provide the ideal of long-term support for this forgotten population. Such groups were developed after the Oakland fire but for individual home fires, such help rarely exists.

Theoretical Considerations

Lindemann's early (1944/1965) work on grief response alerted the health care community to the importance of intervening for a good outcome following disaster. Disaster has been studied exhaustively in the fifty years since his research. Of particular relevance to our study are Murphy's (1984, 1986) studies about survivors of the Mount St. Helen disaster.

Murphy (1984) found that those who had sustained property losses report-ed "greater incidence of negative life events, anger, blame, and financial dissatisfaction than bereaved subjects" (p. 210). Fried (1977), who studied people who had lost their homes because of a relocation project in Eng-land, pointed out the loss of "spatial identity" with the disappearance of familiar spaces of home and neighborhood. In another study of home loss by fire, Keane et al. (1994) reported that the stress of fire victims is of high intensity, and "enduring." In her research, Northrup (1989) posited that disorientation is a normal reaction, and that nurses should support victims rather than hurrying them through to reality-based thinking.

The uniqueness of our theoretical construct is its attention to common social ritual and its connection to victim's comfort. The contrast between rural and urban dwellers is a case in point. In the absence of formal ser-vices, rural residents tend to rituals of neighborly support, so when disas-ter strikes, help is personal and connected to need. However, for crowded urban residents, privacy or disconnectedness with the social world around them allows city dwellers to ignore the plight of others. The end result may be a degree of social isolation. Therefore, for city dwellers, the ritual after a disaster follows this same pattern of "It's-not-my-problem" neglect; paid service workers only partially fill the breach. For inner-city dwellers, the services are often woefully inadequate (Indianapolis fire marshall, Coun-seling Services, personal communication, March 1994).

Conclusions

Often, home fire victims must restructure their lives within a context of ritual-support disconnection. As Glaser (1992) tells us, a grounded the-ory is "readily modifiable" (p. 117) and hence generalizable. Therefore, the concept of restructuring life discovered in this study may have appli-cability for other salient life events for which there are no widespread comforting social rituals. Certainly, the support group concept has been used in these situations as professional rituals to help victim restructure their lives (e.g., "Reach for Recovery," a group to aid survivors of surgi-cal removal of a breast and "Breaking Free," which assists women leav-ing battered-home situations). Fire victims, though, remain uncomforted

(Keane et al., 1994). Programs aimed at awareness could guide the general public in appropriate responses to fire victims.

A nursing intervention study using the support group concept might be a logical next step for adding to our nursing knowledge about home fire victims. Such research might be applicable to several practice areas; for example, mental health/psychiatric nurses could be adept at leading such groups, as could informed community health nurses. In acute care practice, knowledge of the world into which burn victims must return might help these nurses provide care that takes into account the long-term restructuring process and immediate contact with community agencies as well as helping victims understand that relatives might seem distracted. Nursing mentors in school and practice situations might teach these concepts to protégées in mental health, community, and acute care settings. Although other health professionals might be informed by our research, to date they have failed to act.

In her classic work, Maxwell (1979) details the meticulous ways in whic ritual is taught by elders to protégées. In a support group situation, with fire survivors acting as mentors to newer victims of home loss by fire, the passage through the labyrinth of restructuring life after home fire can be eased.

References

Baker, C., Wuest, J. K., & Stern, P. N. (1992). Method slurring: The grounded theory/phenomenology example. *Journal of Advanced Nursing*, 17, 1355–1360.

Bright, M. A. (1990). The therapeutic ritual helping families grow. *Journal of Psychosocial Nursing*, 28, 24–29.

Davis-Floyd, R. (1990). The role of obstetrical rituals in the resolution of cultural anomaly. *Social Science and Medicine*, 31, 175–190.

Farrington, M. A. (1990). The use of rituals in nurse education. *Nursing Times*, 86, 54.

Fried, M. (1977). Grieving for a lost home. In A. Monat & R. Lazarus (Eds.), *Stress and coping. An anthology* (pp. 375–388). New York: Columbia University Press.

Glaser, B. G. (1967). *Theoretical sensitivity.* Mill Valley, CA: Sociology Press.

Glaser, B. G. (1976) *Experts versus laymen: A study of the patsy and the subcontractor.* Mill Valley, CA: Sociology Press.

Glaser, B. G. (1992). *Basic of grounded theory analysis.* Mill Valley, CA: Sociology Press.

Glaser, B. G. (1993). *Examples of grounded theory: A reader.* Mill Valley, CA: Sociology Press.

Glaser, B. G. (1994). *More grounded theory methodology: A reader.* Mill Valley, CA: Sociology Press.

Glaser, B. G., & Strauss, A. L. (1967). *The discovery of grounded theory.* Chicago: Aldine.

Huey, F. L. (1986). Working smart. *American Journal of Nursing*, 86, 679–684.

Hutchinson, S. A. (1983). *Survival practices of rescue workers.* Washington, DC: University Press of America.

Huttmann, B. (1985). Quit wasting time with "nursing rituals." *Nursing*, 15, 34–39.

Jackson, M. M. (1984). From ritual to reason—with a rational approach for the future: An epidemiological perspective. *American Journal of Infection Control*, 12, 213–220.

Keane, A., Pickett, M., Jepson, C., McCorkle, R., & Lowery, B. J. (1994). Psychological distress in survivors of residential fires. *Social Science & Medicine*, 38, 1055–1060.

Kerry, J. (1991). Managing burning: Victims of body and home fire. Unpublished Master's thesis, Dalhousie University, Halifax, Nova Scotia, Canada.

Lindemann, E. (1994). Symptomatology and management of acute grief. In J.

Parad (Ed.), *Crisis intervention: Selected readings* (pp. 7–21). New York: Family Service Association of America. (Original work published 1965).

Maxwell, E. K. (1979). Modeling life: Elder modelers and their protegees. PhD diss., University of California San Francisco. *Dissertation Abstracts International*, 39, 7531A.

Maxwell, E. K. (1993). Expressing awe and fading out. In B. G. Glaser (Ed.), *Examples of grounded theory: A reader* (pp. 163–194). Mill Valley, CA: Sociology Press.

Morse, J. M. (1992). Comfort: The refocusing of nursing care. *Clinical Nursing Research*, 1, 91–113.

Murphy, S. A. (1984). Stress levels and health status of victims of a natural disaster. *Research in Nursing and Health*, 7, 205–215.

Murphy, S. A. (1986). Perceptions of stress, coping and recovery one and three years after a natural disaster. *Issues in Mental Health Nursing*, 8, 63–77.

National Fire Investigation Course Begins. (June 13, 1988). *The Mail Star*, 8.

Northrup, D. T. (1989). Fire loss: Transformative progression from victim to survivor. Unpublished Master's thesis. Dalhousie University, Halifax, Nova Scotia, Canada.

Olien, M. D. (1978). *The human myth*. New York: Harper.

Scheela, R. A. (1992). The remodeling process: A grounded theory study among adult male incest offenders. *Journal of Offender Rehabilitation*, 18, 167–189.

Schmahl, J. (1964). Ritualism in nursing practice. *Nursing Forum*, 3, 74–84.

Stern, P. N. (1980). Grounded theory methodology: Its uses and processes. *Image: Journal of Nursing Scholarship*, 12, 20–23.

Stern, P. N. (1985). Using grounded theory in nursing research. In M. Leininger (Ed.), *Qualitative research methods in nursing* (pp. 149–160). New York: Grune & Stratton.

Stern, P. N. (1991). Are counting and coding a cappella appropriate in qualitative research? In J. M. Morse (Eds.), *Qualitative nursing research: A contemporary dialogue* (pp. 147–162). Newbury Park, CA: Sage.

Stern, P. N. (1994). Eroding grounded theory. In J. M. Morse (Ed.), *Critical issues in qualitative inquiry* (pp. 212–223). Newbury Park, CA: Sage.

Stern, P. N., Allen, L. M., & Moxley, P. A. (1982). The nurse as grounded theorist: History, processes and uses. *The Review Journal of Philosophy and Social Science*, 7, 200–215.

Strauss, A. L. (1987). *Qualitative analysis for social scientists*. New York: Cambridge University Press.

Walker, V. (1967). *Nursing and ritualistic practice*. New York: Macmillan.

Welsh, M., & Ford, P. (1989a). Rituals in nursing: We always do it this way. *Nursing Times*, 85, 26–35.

Welsh, M., & Ford, P. (1989b). Rituals in nursing: It can't hurt that much. *Nursing Times*, 85, 35–38.

Welsh, M., & Ford, P. (1989c). Rituals in nursing: A day in the ward. *Nursing Times*, 85, 45–48.

Wolf, Z. (1988). Nursing rituals. *The Canadian Journal of Nursing Research*, 20, 59–69.

Wolin, S. J. & Bennett, L. A. (1984). Family rituals. *Family Process*, 23, 401–420.

Dialogue: The Ethics of Interviewing

Hi, I'm a doctoral student. First of all, I want to thank all of you for such an insightful day. Here's my question: I kind of loved the authors of constructivist grounded theory and I tried to get insight into something of the methodological challenges for a psychologist like myself, just because it's new, and I don't know of any writing on that and I'm just looking for insight or your opinions. ...

Kathy: I can give some advice, and you can take it for what its worth. ...

At first when you revisit what has gone before in your research, you're open to so much more to what's going on now. Often you don't know what's going on and you gently try to find out. And sometimes, with people that I've been with for a long time, the personal comes first before the research project. So I know their voices and they give cues that they want to open up about something, so then we'll talk about it.

I'll give you an example. At the beginning of an interview, a woman sat down and said, "I was raped." I let her talk—I did not press. I just listened for a long time and she told her story. I really didn't think it was appropriate for me to ask her in-depth interview questions about it for a couple of reasons, including that it wasn't the topic of my research. So there was no dialogue between us and I just didn't feel comfortable going beyond what she wanted to say. But I certainly wanted her to say anything she wished, and if you have an attitude of openness, people pick up on it and they'll tell you the things that you never expected.

One of the things that's so wonderful about doing research is that you learn so much that you never anticipated, and to be willing to be with them to hear what they want to say may prove to be significant.

I'm also very concerned about premature analytical publishing, and so I prefer to leave things analytically open for awhile. But my job situation is such that I may not get to coding something that was done very recently but I'll go back to it. And I also want to tell you to that when you go back to data, you see things you never anticipated. You had no idea about the world of your participants earlier or something else comes up that had not occurred to you before. So that's another thing—write memos relatively early, but know they are incomplete and they are open to correction. Keep writing and developing them, or just put them in a pile and stop using that set of memos until later.

Barbara: One of the things that I've seen students struggle with is when someone who is interviewed is incredibly open, and an awful lot has been disclosed. We don't talk about this a lot, but I think there's some work that needs to be done at the end of the interview. I think it's not a good idea to just get up and walk out. There is some work that needs to be done. You cannot leave a person who has fallen apart without putting them back together.

Kathy: That's a very good point. I tell my students that when they are doing an interview, that they have to allow for time to have tea or coffee with the person. They have got to allow for time to bring their interviewee back to a normal level of conversation. I think it's unethical not to, and leaving the person in a vulnerable place is simply unacceptable.

Phyllis: Well, I couldn't agree more.

5. Dimensional Analysis

Barbara Bowers and Leonard Schatzman

Dimensional analysis is an approach to research developed by Leonard Schatzman, a student and later colleague of Anselm Strauss. This chapter is presented as a brief introduction to dimensional analysis. A more in-depth treatment of the approach will be described in greater detail in a subsequent publication.

This chapter will provide an overview of:

1. the context and development of dimensional analysis, including personal biographical information about Dr. Leonard Schatzman, specifically as it has influenced the development of dimensional analysis;

2. the relationship between dimensional analysis and grounded theory;

3. the contributions of dimensional analysis in regard to teaching analysis and learning to conduct analysis;

4. a discussion of natural analysis as universal form of human reasoning integral to the development of personhood; and

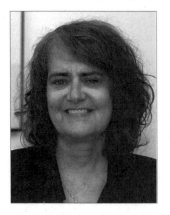

5. the relationship between natural analysis and dimensional analysis.

Unlike other versions of grounded theory, dimensional analysis is still taught primarily as an oral tradition, passed along largely from teacher to student and colleague to colleague. Although Schatzman has published little on dimensional analysis, his 1991 chapter on dimensional analysis (Schatzman, 1991) and several articles published by former students

(Caron & Bowers, 2000; Kools et al., 1996) provide some introduction to the method. Many other studies using dimensional analysis have been published by Schatzman's students (Bowers, 1987, 1988, 1989, 1996; Bowers & Becker, 1992; Bowers, Esmond, & Canales, 1999; Bowers, Esmond, & Jacobson, 2000, 2003; Bowers, Fibich, & Jacobson, 2001; Bowers, Lauring, & Jacobson, 2001; Bowers et al., 2006; Brown & Olshansky, 1997; Kools, 1997, 1999; Kools, Gilliss, & Tong, 1999; Kools & Kennedy, 2002; Kools & Spiers, 2002; Kools et al., 1996; Kools, et al., 2002; McCarthy, 2003a, 2003b; McCarthy et al., 2004; Liang & Olshansky, 2005; Olshansky, 1987a, 1987b, 1993a, 1993b, 2005; Watson, Kieckhefer, & Olshansky, 2006) and, in turn, by their students (Caron & Bowers, 2003; DeVore & Bowers, 2006; Hamilton & Bowers, 2005, in press; Lutz & Bowers, 2005; Lutz et al., 2003; Norton & Bowers, 2001), providing some additional insights about the research method.

Personal Biography and Association with Anselm Strauss

As with all intellectual traditions, personal biography and social circumstances played an important role in the development of dimensional analysis. Specifically, Schatzman's long association with Anselm Strauss is reflected in the development of dimensional analysis. Schatzman began his association with Strauss when he became Strauss's first graduate student at Indiana University, in 1946. From Anselm Strauss, Schatzman learned about research and developed both a passion for Chicago School Sociology and a strong sociological worldview. As he watched Strauss and other field researchers collect data and write monographs, he began to wonder what actually happened between the selection of a research question and the final monograph, what was involved in the analysis, how did the researcher actually "do" analysis, how did researchers learn to do research? How did perspectives and conceptual commitments held by researchers influence the research they did? Indeed, how does someone come to do analysis in a way that is similar to colleagues in the same discipline yet different from those in other disciplines? Analysis was a mysterious process. As Schatzman recalls, during his early graduate years he asked Strauss for a description or definition of analysis, an explanation of what analysis was and how analysis was done.

Strauss responded to Schatzman's questions about analysis as many mentors did then and still do today. He said, "Watch me. Work with me.

Read monographs extensively and you will see." Like most students, Schatzman followed that advice and eventually did see and was able to do analysis on his own. By the end of his graduate program, he saw and understood as a sociologist, with a sociological eye (Hughes, 1984). Although he was largely satisfied with this new ability, he did not then realize that Chicago School theory was the perspective that guided his understanding and framed his analyses (i.e., that he was "theory driven" although not explicitly so, not yet identifying the theoretical framework in his work). And despite being able to conduct research, to do analysis (through received theory–Chicago School sociology), he was still unable to indicate the steps he was using in the process of analysis. The process of analysis remained a mystery. This continuing mystery stayed a significant force in the development of dimensional analysis.

From this early time, Schatzman was interested in the nature of analysis in general, although was never really interested in developing a research methodology. After three years of teaching sociology, Schatzman spent three years working with Strauss and Rue Bucher, another former student of Strauss, on a study of psychiatry, psychiatric professions, treatment philosophies, and institutions (Strauss et al., 1964). In retrospect, Schatzman has thought about how smoothly this research went, without any explicit plan for analysis or understanding about what analysis actually was. What the researchers shared, of course, was a sociological view of the world and an accessible set of sociological concepts to use in their analysis. So, although their analysis continued quite nicely, quite intuitively, without ever having to figure out what analysis was, Schatzman continued to puzzle over the nature of analysis.

Toward the end of the psychiatry study, Strauss was invited to the University of California at San Francisco (UCSF) School of Nursing to encourage and support faculty to develop research skills, conduct research, and publish. Strauss negotiated an agreement that allowed him to bring a small faculty along with him to support faculty development to teach graduate students to do research and eventually to assist in the development of a doctoral program in nursing. Through this arrangement, Schatzman and a few other sociologists joined the nursing faculty at UCSF.

Schatzman recalls the bright and eager nursing students coming to UCSF to learn to do research who would invariably ask the same question Schatzman asked when he began his work at Indiana: How does one actually "do" analysis? The students were asking him questions such as "What exactly happens in analysis?" "What is analysis and how is it done?" "How can I learn to do analysis?" and "How do I know when I am doing analysis? Or doing it correctly?" Schatzman found himself giving the same response that he had been given by his mentor, Strauss, and that so many students learning qualitative analysis still hear today: "Work with me for a while and you will see." He found this answer unsatisfying, but it had worked for him and he reasoned that it would work for his students. But the mystery of analysis remained and continued to occupy him.

Although Strauss and Schatzman continued to work together, their research partnership lasted primarily into the mid-1960s, when Strauss began to work much more closely with Barney Glaser. After that, the collaboration between Strauss and Schatzman was primarily in relation to students for whom they served together on dissertation committees, although they also continued to read and discuss each other's work.

Strauss's work with Glaser on *The Discovery of Grounded Theory* in 1967 (Glaser & Strauss, 1967), and his 1987 publication on *Qualitative Analysis for Social Scientists* reflected Strauss's ongoing devotion to developing the grounded theory method, leading them in somewhat different directions, intellectually. During this time, Schatzman was still primarily interested in understanding analysis in general, now involving an effort to produce a general theory of analysis. In the late 1970s and early 1980s, Strauss was being pressured to explain what he did and how he conducted analysis in response to both his students and many other researchers who found his work theoretically rich while clearly reflecting the social world or phenomenon that was the object of study. This culminated in his *Qualitative Analysis for Social Scientists* (1987). Schatzman, on the other hand, was still primarily interested understanding analysis in general, in developing a "general theory of analysis."

As Strauss's work on grounded theory evolved, Strauss and Schatzman had many conversations about the direction the method was taking. Schatzman was intrigued with grounded theory, thinking this might finally lead to an understanding of the nature of analysis or even provide a theory of analysis for qualitative research. He and Strauss had many conversations about grounded theory during this time. Strauss acknowledges Schatzman's influence on the development of his thinking about analysis, in particular about dimensionalizing that Strauss describes as an important aspect of open coding, in his 1987 book on *Qualitative Analysis for Social Scientists*, and about the early versions of the conditional matrix. The relevant point here is that Schatzman's ideas about analysis were largely generated out of these discussions with Strauss in the late 1960s to mid-1970s. After that, there was little interaction between them about research analysis.

Dimensional Analysis: Convergences with Grounded Theory

Although dimensional analysis developed at least in part as a response to what Schatzman saw as limitations of early grounded theory, there is considerable overlap between them. The nature and extent of the similarities between dimensional analysis and grounded theory depend to some extent on which version of grounded theory is considered in the comparison. This discussion is based on grounded theory as reflected in *Qualitative Analysis for Social Scientists* (Strauss, 1987).

Grounded theory (à la Strauss) and dimensional analysis have similar intellectual foundations. That is, they are both firmly rooted in the Chicago School of Sociology, informed by symbolic interaction, and initially developed by sociologists with clear commitments to both an interactionist worldview and the questions generally addressed by sociologists, particularly those related to social process. At different times, Schatzman describes dimensional analysis as developed "in the wake of grounded theory," as "generally informed by the core ideas and practices of grounded theory," as "an alternative approach to grounding theory in data," and as "philosophically, following the work of Strauss." Dimensional analysis, like grounded theory, was designed for the generation of theory directly from data. This is in contrast to much research, qualitative and quantitative, that is theory directed or theory tested.

Dimensional Analysis: Schatzman's Response to Grounded Theory

Schatzman was initially quite excited about the power of comparative analysis that the grounded theory method offered, seeing grounded theory as having distinct advantages over theory-controlled analysis. However, he felt that something was missing. Specifically, as he watched the development of the grounded theory method and worked with students using the method to conduct their research, he began to see that, despite the usefulness of comparison, the method seemed to minimize the complexity and the subtlety of analytic reasoning and failed to acknowledge the wider range of analytic processes that, in addition to comparison, were involved in analysis. So, although appreciating the power of constant comparison, Schatzman began searching for an understanding of analysis that was broader than grounded theory and acknowledged and could accommodate both the wider range of analytic processes and greater complexity of analytic operations required to conduct analysis of any sort.

Schatzman first began to realize why comparative analysis as a focus for operations was not adequate to describe and to teach analysis as he worked with students who were trying to do qualitative analysis in the context of grounded theory. As he listened to students describe what they were doing, he was hearing clear and repeated descriptions of many other analytic processes that were integral to their analysis.

In 1973, Schatzman wrote his field research text, which included a chapter devoted to analysis. The text was intended to be a collaboration. However, as Schatzman completed the first draft, it became clear to both Strauss and Schatzman that this work reflected a clear departure between grounded theory and the direction Schatzman was taking. Continuing to puzzle over the nature of analysis, he hoped that dealing with it as part of the field research text might somehow assist him to develop a position or perspective on analysis that would be suitable to any qualitative research problem. Initially believing that he had failed in this effort but with Strauss's urging, he published the book (Schatzman & Strauss, 1973). Still without a theory of analysis, he continued until 1975 to help individual doctorate students who were using the grounded theory method to complete their research work. Returning later to this text, Schatzman saw clearly the beginnings of dimensional analysis.

In 1975, the dean of the School of Nursing asked Schatzman to teach a course on qualitative research for a dozen or so students in the Master's program who needed some credits in research. He was told that the students were clinically focused and not really interested in research and that on graduation, they would be seeking clinical positions. Faced with the task of teaching qualitative research, including describing analysis to students who did not have a clear understanding of analysis in general, he asked them to discuss what considerations they would use to decide from among several job offers which one they would select.

The students indicated a number of considerations in lay terms bearing principally on professional perspective. Schatzman interpreted these as expressing clinical specialty, philosophical compatibility, and role autonomy.

As Schatzman encouraged students to identify the criteria they would use to consider and ultimately select their first nursing position, he noticed how they were selecting some dimensions while ignoring others. Schatzman observed the nursing students as they conjured dimensions, seeing some as highly valued whereas others were seen as of little relevance. For example, they identified model of care as very important; type of care or the particular unit was viewed as much less important. They described patient population as somewhat important, but size and appearance of the building were not important at all. Schatzman then asked for additional considerations and when none were forthcoming, he volunteered such considerations as salary, workload, and work shift. The students responded with exclamations of "Naturally," "Obviously," or "Sure."

As Schatzman considered how the students were conjuring dimensions, he offered a few that might have been relevant to other similar analytic process such as selecting an apartment or selecting a part time position before graduation. These dimensions were summarily dismissed by students as irrelevant. For example, working with a friend might have been one of the most important considerations for a part-time position during graduate school. Geographic location might be one of the most important dimensions of selecting an apartment, especially for students with limited time and transportation alternatives but might be only somewhat relevant for taking a first nursing position.

Students were obviously attributing greater value to some dimensions than to others. So although they were clearly engaged in comparative analysis of nursing positions, comparison alone could not account for the positions they might consider or accept. Their comparisons proceeded on the basis of prior assumptions and understandings about the nature and variable importance of these considerations. The possibility of comparison and the nature of the comparison relied on their ability to call out and evaluate particular dimensions. Those not known or not identified were obviously not included in their comparative analysis. Schatzman concluded that although the ability to call out or designate and attribute value to dimensions is implicit in comparative analysis, these other analytic processes were also necessary for comparative analysis but had not actually been identified as part of or necessary for comparative analysis in grounded theory or other qualitative research. This failure to explicitly recognize these other processes made teaching or learning qualitative research, including grounded theory, much more difficult than it needed to be. In addition, the failure to acknowledge these other analytic processes was at least a partial explanation for the mysterious nature of analysis.

It was then that Schatzman "discovered" dimensional analysis. He concluded that he had tapped an important aspect of natural analysis and that considerations are, in fact, dimensions of experience—in this case nurses' experiences—and constitute the wherewithal to construct, analyze, and define situations (see Schatzman, 1991).

Enjoying a reputation as a master teacher and someone always accessible to students, many students visited Schatzman to gain insight into what Strauss (and other faculty) was telling them to do and how to proceed with their analysis. As Schatzman helped students learn to conduct a grounded theory analysis, it became increasingly clear that many other analytic processes were involved in analysis. As Schatzman interacted with these students, many he advised jointly with Strauss, he became increasingly dissatisfied with the "procedures" or operations of grounded theory and the limitations of constant comparative analysis. So, although appreciating the power of comparative analysis, Schatzman continued to develop his ideas about dimensional analysis.

Schatzman's thoughts about the importance of these other analytic processes were also supported by his encounters with students who were working with Strauss and others and who were having great difficulty learning to do grounded theory. These students would sometimes come to Schatzman for help in identifying the operations involved in grounded theory analysis. They sought assistance in figuring out how to proceed with their analysis, having great difficulty understanding the process, how to get started, and how the conceptual categories were generated. The students were focused on comparing and comparative analysis but were finding it difficult to proceed with their analysis using that single analytic tool to conduct their analysis. This operation, comparison, was simply not sufficient for them to conduct analysis.

Schatzman concluded that research analysis involves a range of analytic processes, only one of which is comparative analysis. Some of the other analytic processes, necessary in conducting research analysis, include:

- Conjuring, calling up dimensions (characteristics). This conjuring process often proceeds unproblematically and invisibly in qualitative analysis. The impact of other analytic procedures on the conjuring process is generally not taken account of, proceeding as if the identified dimensions were the only possible dimensions.

- Assigning relative value to each of the dimensions considered. This is the process of determining which dimensions would be viewed as irrelevant, determining which dimensions are nothing and nonsense as well as those that rise to the level of relevance or even salience. This analytic process is engaged in by analysts but is not made visible to others or even to the self. Attributions of value are embedded (albeit often without acknowledgement) in personal and professional biography, and operate to screen and select dimensions that are considered or "identified" as inherent in the situation.

- Inferring, making inferences about dimensions conjured. Although comparison facilitates analysis of dimensions conjured and selected, comparison relies on the researcher assuming relationship among dimensions and assuming relevance or irrelevance of those dimensions.

A second observation Schatzman made was the focus of grounded theory on identifying *a* basic social process and doing so quite early in the process of analysis. He saw the consequences of this as a premature focus on logically deduced or logically conjured comparisons, taking the research outside the data, developing theory from dimensions that were external to the data, ultimately limiting the researcher's understanding of the phenomenon being studied. Using comparison, comparative analysis, which facilitated or stimulated conceptualizing at this early point, increased the distance between the researcher and the data. This was inconsistent with grounded theory's explicit purpose of developing theory from empirically generated data. Schatzman reasoned that focusing on "what all is involved" in the data, rather than a single, basic social process, would prevent the premature closure that would result from early comparisons and would ultimately minimize the distancing between researcher and the data.

So, Schatzman reasoned, taking a broader approach to analysis (as more than comparative analysis), asking "what *all* is involved," would likely generate a wide range of dimensions related to the phenomenon under study, avoiding early theoretical closure, leading the researcher to a much fuller and more complex range of dimensions and properties before undertaking analysis and engaging in comparative analysis. This broader approach to dimensionalizing, he believed, was necessary to handle the complexity of social life. Following this logic, conceptualizing too early would result in a much narrower, less rich view of the phenomenon. This meant that staying open to "what all is involved" would lead to a richer and more grounded understanding of a phenomenon. Consequently, it is the job of the researcher to encourage informants to designate concepts, calling out dimensions and properties, to develop a rich and comprehensive bank of dimensions generated from the informant.

This view of analysis is reflected in the advice that Strauss and Schatzman gave to their students when asked "How long do I stay focused on my data before I begin to compare, to logically deduce possibilities?" (Strauss, 1987). Students working with Strauss were generally directed to begin comparative analysis immediately (Strauss, 1987), that the analyst was engaged in comparison right from the beginning. Schatzman took a different approach, suggesting that comparative analysis should be delayed until a larger bank of dimensions had been identified in the data.

Dimensional Analysis: A New Path

Dimensional analysis is committed to an expansive, early process of identifying and designating dimensions and their properties to expand the analyst's understanding of the object of study; the relevance, complexity, and possibilities of any dimension can generally only be determined by understanding the perspective from which it is viewed. Perspective both limits and directs analysis, whether everyday analysis or research analysis. Perspective not only determines the selection and designation or dimensions, it also directs their organization or their relationships to one another. Left relatively unaddressed in grounded theory as well as in most other qualitative research, even today, was the question of researcher perspective and how perspective (commitment, discipline, or personal biography) was embedded in the analysis, guiding the identification and designation of dimensions, the direction of comparative analysis (and consequently the direction of conceptualizing), and the organization of dimensions (theory development).

Schatzman suggested that perspective needed to be viewed in a much more complex way than was generally the case in qualitative analysis, that a more sophisticated understanding of how both operated in analysis was vital. His experience with students working on grounded theory studies at UCSF, along with his reading of texts in qualitative research, suggested that there was pervasive insufficient recognition of the role that perspective plays in analysis, either the researcher's analysis of the data or the informants' representation (analysis) of the phenomenon being studied. That is, researchers were not recognizing the role that perspective played in the conjuring and organizing of dimensions offered by informants and they were not recognizing how their own perspectives as researchers or analysts were operating in considering, valuing, and selecting concepts they determined to be relevant. Schatzman also reasoned that there were multiple perspectives to consider during analysis, that informants might take different perspectives depending on the context, that a "good" analysis would include more than a single perspective, and that it would, in fact, seek to identify multiple perspectives and understand how those perspectives influenced the stories they told. Schatzman's description of nursing students considering offers of employment illustrates how perspective operates in analysis.

When asked to think about employment offers and to determine which offers might be "the best" ones, nursing students initially provided reasons (explanations for selection of particular dimensions) that were oriented to a classroom situation, answering from a professional perspective, talking about vision and philosophy. Being asked by a professor, seeing other professionals and the professor as audience, students answered from a professional perspective. However, when students were asked about several dimensions of work that no one had had previously considered (i.e., work routine: pay, work shift and shift rotation, modes of transportation, safety of setting, distance, and parking), the students uniformly responded with "Of course," "Naturally," "Sure." Although these dimensions were not conjured up in a "professional" perspective, they were perspectives that were easily accessed by students, albeit with differing levels of relevance. Using a professional perspective in response to the classroom situation, students with limited incomes and large debts might actually use a different perspective when selecting a position, making pay, transportation costs, and opportunity for overtime more central dimensions in their analysis. This simple example begins to illustrate the coexistence of multiple perspectives, the emerging and shifting salience of a particular perspective in response to context, and the resulting consequences of perspective for selection, designation, and organization of dimensions.

When students were offered a new perspective—practical rather than professional—they were led to a new set of dimensions to consider and responded to the question from that new angle or perspective. For at least some, this led to a new conclusion about the job they would select. Schatzman recognized that initially they had answered his question from the perspective of a professional in an academic setting, and their responses were crafted from that perspective. However, when they adopted another perspective, one that was just as real for them in their decision-making, the response or conclusion could be quite different. What was important both for understanding analysis and the development of research operations or methods was the realization that "humans are doomed to be selective," to take a perspective on problems, to see from a standpoint. In fact, informants in a research project can only tell their story from a perspective, granted at different times possibly from different perspectives, but never without a perspective. The relevance for research analysis is that researchers can only conduct an analysis from a perspective. Analysis cannot be done without a perspective.

At the time (in the 1970s), perspective and how (or even whether) it operated in analysis was receiving little attention in qualitative research, including grounded theory studies, although there have certainly been important discussions about perspective, including researcher biography, since then. There was recognition that ideology influences the determination of relevance, salience, and irrelevance. However, awareness of the power of perspective did not seem to extend to questions about how the perspectives of disciplines and individual researchers (unproblematically) operated to select and limit the dimensions included in any analysis, to determine which dimensions were deemed to be of some value or "of interest" to the researcher. Schatzman saw the influence of perspective most clearly in the differences between analyses of nursing students and students in sociology.

Students in sociology came to analysis with sociological concepts; nursing students came with concerns about clinical questions. Their lenses (perspectives) were different. The dimensions conjured by nursing students differed from those of their sociological-minded colleagues. This difference was often understood by sociology faculty as being less sophisticated analysis rather than as analysis generated from a different perspective. Failing to tease out how perspective was directing the gaze of student researchers made it difficult for students to understand how to improve their analysis or even why it was seen as lacking. It also prevented students and their advisors from seeing that, at least some of the time, sociological concepts were deemed to be more acceptable, reflecting more sophisticated analysis than were clinical concepts.

The recognition that perspective is always operating also raised questions about the notion of emergence in qualitative research. Recognizing that what "emerges" from data is dependent on both the perspective of the informant and the perspective of the researcher, the notion of emergence as unproblematic discovery in much qualitative research, even today, is an insufficient, even misleading explanation of analysis, failing to account for the range of analytic processes that lead to selection and organization of dimensions. Schatzman was concerned that the failure to take perspective into account was responsible for the common mistaking of "received" conception and prior assumptions for discovered truth.

Recognition/Recall

Recognition/recall involves the ability to find a designation for the object of interest or for its dimensions. It is the designation of dimensions from data, which are guided or determined by prior assumptions and perspectives of the analyst. Anthropologists will find culture in their data; psychologists will find motivation or other psychological constructs; more ideologically informed analysts will find inequality and oppression. Researchers learn theories, conceptual frameworks, core disciplinary concepts, and acquire the vocabularies that these concepts are embedded in. These concepts suggest to students and other members of the discipline what they should be observing in the field and how to translate data into knowledge, thus directing their endeavors and their discoveries. Once novices take on the perspective of the discipline, bringing this perspective to their analysis, they no longer need a definition of analysis. They have the concepts they need to find what is relevant in the data they generate. This is often mistaken for emergence that is not beholden to any theoretical perspective, as pure discovery. In this instance, discovery is rendered an organizational or labeling problem rather than a conceptual one.

In Schatzman's view, scientific research and analysis are taught in academic institutions by experts in the various disciplines, both quantitative and qualitative, using analytic tools that are grounded in a perspective, with their own vocabularies. In other words, the processes for analyzing substance are hidden in the vocabulary and knowledge of each science, discipline, or perspective.

Analysis is different. Analysis occurs when a problematic situation is encountered, when recognition and recall are not sufficient to understand what is going on. Analysis, at least theory-generating work, allows for competing explanations or definitions and must always be done from a perspective. An important question for researchers wanting to learn the experiences of research informants is whether the perspective operating to select and organize dimensions is that of the informants or that of the researcher (and the researcher's discipline). In daily life, recognition/recall is an appropriate and efficient way to understand the world and the things around us. In research, recognition/recall can block analysis, stopping the conjuring of dimensions or the seeking of new dimensions and properties. It essentially precludes transparency in the conjuring, valuing, and selecting of dimensions to include in the analysis and the decision about their importance.

Learning to Do Analysis

One of the most intriguing aspects of Schatzman's work is his proposal that the operations involved in research analysis and the analysis we all engage in everyday to solve mundane problems, to figure things out, to explain and evaluate the things in our daily lives, are essentially the same. Schatzman believed that the failure to understand this, and to perpetuate a belief that research analysis is fundamentally different than natural analysis, that students come to the research process as novices in "doing analysis," is a major source of difficulty for students learning to become researchers. Descriptions of analysis in qualitative research texts, including grounded theory, failed to relate the analytic strategies used by researchers to those used naturally.

According to Schatzman, research analysis was and is discussed by most teachers of qualitative research as requiring an order of thinking, a quality of thinking that is quite different from the thinking we engage in during more mundane activities. Although there are few descriptions of how to do analysis, there seems to be a general belief that analysis is something that novices need to be taught. That is, students do not come to research programs with a sophisticated knowledge of how to do analysis.

In reviewing texts on qualitative research, Schatzman observed that many of these texts, especially those written within a discipline, offered the novice researcher concepts that were core to that discipline, as sufficient components or structures for analysis; that is, providing theory or perspective relevant to the discipline was offered as the tool to conduct analysis. This meant that the concepts of the discipline would be brought to the data, not derived from the data, but presented as analysis.

This observation became important for Schatzman's ideas about analysis, as it suggested that the researcher's prior perspective leads to "recognition" of the dimensions relevant to that perspective, and that the process is experienced as "discovery." That is, researchers use what Schatzman calls recognition/recall rather than any formal analysis grounded in the data, to derive theory from data or to "discover" what is in the data. So, when looking at how theorizing is actually done, he realized that sociologists generally theorized by bringing the concepts of sociology to the interpretation.

Other texts on qualitative research, those that did not offer theory or conceptual frameworks from a particular perspective, generally provided little to guide the novice about how to actually do analysis, what to do with data. When guidance was offered about the analysis or interpreting process, it was largely procedural rather than analytic. For example, readers were instructed to read and reread their notes, to immerse themselves in the data or the field. This is similar to the advice Schatzman had received from his advisor: Watch, listen, read monographs, and immerse yourself. The lack of attention to what is occurring *analytically* often reflects recognition/recall, when researchers bring concepts to the analysis, use them to determine relevance of dimensions, organize the dimensions according to the discipline's perspective, and experience the process as discovery. In either case, the actual process of analysis or interpretation is invisible, even to the researchers. Without understanding the processes by which an interpretation is actually made, the experience will continue to be inaccessible and mysterious.

Variations in analysis and findings occur as a consequence of who is doing the analysis, as people have private commitments, interests, sensitivities and tolerances, and ways of seeing, weighing, and choosing options. Ideas and findings are competitive. All social disciplines have advocates of differing perspectives and more than one perspective on the reality of its substance. Every analyst conjures and gathers his or her own considerations, weighs and values each, and configures them into a pattern or story that expresses a logic and sequence.

Making perspectives and their operation in the "emergent" theory transparent would require that perspectives are recognized, disclosed, and tracked. This would result in a higher level of researcher self-consciousness about and acceptance of greater responsibility for the substance of the analysis than is generally the case.

Natural Analysis

Schatzman's longstanding question about the nature of analysis led to his close observation of how we all analyze every day, solving mundane problems and figuring things out. Schatzman observed that all analysis, not just research analysis, requires a property of thinking that he refers to as "dimensionality." He suggests that human intelligence dimensionalizes experience and constructs or defines situations dimensionally, which is necessary to understand complexity. Dimensionalizing allows us to see things in their complexity, to discriminate among them, and to compare one thing to another. Any description of something involves an identification of its dimensions and properties.

Schatzman sees analysis as basic to all human understanding and interaction. Analysis is "natural," learned early in life, and practiced "constantly in experience." As he pointed out to students he worked with, everyone arrives in graduate school with a sophisticated ability to engage in analysis. The nursing students looking for jobs were analyzing the options, attributing value, selecting from among the possibilities. They were analyzing the situation, analyzing from a perspective. Humans born into a social system learn its language and culture and become socialized. In that process, children begin to develop a conception of self. The child learns many designations and evaluates them as good, bad, and irrelevant, learning to designate and to organize behavior around designations. The child is then expected to continue both explaining actions and organizing actions around designations and their evaluations. As this ability becomes more sophisticated, the child begins to conjure, sort, and select considerations for inclusion in their "definitions of the situation." These understandings are informed, in increasingly complex ways, by perspective. The child learns to take into account the perspectives and the logic of the audience to which the interaction is directed, to take the role of the other, to create an explanation that will be plausible to "the other." In any event, the scholar or street person who expresses an understanding to others on any topic must speak to the logic of others as audience and then await the others' acceptance or rejection of the assertion. Validity is in the eye of the beholder and is inherent in the vocabulary and logic applied to the explanation.

These observations led to Schatzman's exploration of the similarities between natural analysis, what we all do every day, and research analysis. This aspect of his work is significant for the teaching and learning of research analysis in particular. His conclusion was that research analysis is similar in kind to natural analysis. They are simply informed by different perspectives, guided by attention to different audiences, but in terms of the analytic tools and the logic used, they are essentially the same.

The example he often uses to illustrate this is the problem of explaining the actions of a woman sitting all day in front of a bank of slot machines. An evangelist tells us that the devil made her gamble; a Marxist would say it was the capitalist system that enticed and exploited the woman; a geneticist might hypothesize the existence of a gene related to addiction. All three positions adhere to a logic of cause and provide internally consistent logics, verbalizing their explanations in different languages, from different perspectives, using different a priori logics and vocabularies. Thus, depending on who is listening, each explanation will or will not be sensible, rational, or ridiculous.

Being impressed by what he saw as the universality of analysis in human reasoning and the tools to engage in analysis, Schatzman concluded that it would be quite useful, in teaching analysis to novices, to disabuse them of the beliefs that:

1. lay capacity for analysis is different from and inferior to scientific analysis. Rather, Schatzman sees research analysis as itself a natural development, a subtype of ordinary human reasoning, suggesting that scientific research is a modified form of lay analysis, not different in kind; and

2. qualitative analysis is generally quite independent of theory, that something can be discovered without a theory or perspective to guide the inquiry. As Schatzman concluded, researchers and audiences barely see, or don't see, the relationship between knowledge and disciplinary perspective and their "discoveries."

Making visible the link between analysis involved in research and that involved in common interpretative acts, Schatzman believed, could have the effect of demystifying research analysis, making analysis of any kind more transparent and more amenable to instruction than "Watch me and you will pick it up." This view essentially renders analysis not only transparent but also recognizable as a common human skill, and therefore comfortably familiar to students "learning to do analysis."

Dimensional analysis, then, is a fundamental component of natural, everyday analysis as well as research analysis. It is concerned with how someone comes to "define the situation" (be it researcher or informant), with making explicit the analytic processes involved in the interpreting, discovering, or constructing processes. It keeps the question of perspective in the forefront and seeks to make transparent the things that are often, in qualitative research, not considered explicitly or at all by the analysts engaged in analysis or the audiences.

Dimensional analysis shares with grounded theory a commitment to generating theory directly from data. It recognizes and integrates the perspectives of the researcher as well as those of the informants or subjects of research. Dimensional analysis seeks to make transparent the analytic processes used by researchers as they conduct their analysis. The methodology directs the researcher to remain open to what informants have to say, seeking to identify a rich bank of dimensions prior to beginning analysis, preventing early conceptual closure. As a research method, dimensional analysis interferes with the tendency for qualitative researchers to label concepts early in analysis, engaging in recognition recall, thereby blocking the development of rich and grounded theory. Although dimensional analysis shares much with the other grounded theory methods, it differs in its assumptions about the centrality and timing of comparative analysis and differs from some of the grounded theory methods in not supporting the search for a single, basic social process, rather seeking to learn "what all is involved," thus recognizing the complexity of social life. Finally, dimensional analysis explicitly recognizes and embraces the sophisticated analytic skills that are used by all of us in our daily lives, adapting these skills to the research enterprise.

References

Bowers, B. J. (1987). Intergenerational caregiving: Adult caregivers and their aging parents. *Advances in Nursing Science*, 9(2), 20–31.

Bowers, B. J. (1988). Family perceptions of care in nursing homes. *The Gerontologist*, 28(3), 361–368.

Bowers, B. J. (1989). Grounded theory: From conceptualization to research process. In B. Sarter (Ed.), *Paths to knowledge: Innovative research methods in nursing* (pp. 33–58). New York: National League of Nursing.

Bowers, B. J. (1996). *The relationship between staffing and quality in long-term care facilities.* Report to the 105th U.S. Congress, Subcommittee on Health: Appropriateness of Minimum Nurse Staffing Ratios.

Bowers, B. J. & Becker, M. (1992). Nurse aides in nursing homes: The relationship between organization and quality. *The Gerontologist*, 32(3), 360–366.

Bowers, B. J., Esmond, S., & Canales, M. (1999). Approaches to case management supervision. *Administration in Social Work*, 23(1), 29–49.

Bowers, B. J., Esmond, S., & Jacobson, N. (2000). The relationship between staffing and quality in long-term care facilities: Exploring the views of nurse aides. *Journal of Nursing Care Quality*, 14(4), 55–64.

Bowers, B. J., Esmond, S., & Jacobson, N. (2003). Turnover reinterpreted: CNAs talk about why they leave. *Journal of Gerontological Nursing*, 29(3), 36–43.

Bowers, B. J., Esmond, S. L., Norton, S., & Holloway, E. (2006). The consumer/provider relationship as care quality mediator. In S. Kunkel & V. Wellin (Eds.), *Consumer voice and choice in long-term care* (ch. 10). New York: Springer.

Bowers, B. J., Fibich, B., & Jacobson, N. (2001). Care as service, care as relating, care as comfort: Understanding nursing home residents' perceptions of quality. *The Gerontologist*, 41(4), 539–545.

Bowers, B. J., Lauring, C., & Jacobson, N. (2001). How nurses manage time and work in long-term care facilities. *Journal of Advanced Nursing*, 33(4), 484–491.

Brown, M. A. & Olshansky, E. F. (1997). From limbo to legitimacy: A theoretical model of the transition to the primary care nurse practitioner role. *Nursing Research*, 46 (1), 46–51.

Caron, C. & Bowers, B. J. (2000). Methods and application of dimensional analysis: A contribution to concept and knowledge development in nursing. In B. L. Rodgers & K. A. Knafl (Eds.), *Concept development in nursing, foundations, techniques and applications* (pp. 285–319). Philadelphia: W.B. Saunders Co.

Caron, C. D. & Bowers, B. J. (2003). Deciding whether to continue, share or relinquish caregiving: Caregiver views. *Qualitative Health Research*, 13(9), 1252–1271.

DeVore, D. J. & Bowers, B. J. (2006). Childcare for children with disabilities: Families search for specialized care and cooperative childcare partnerships. *Infants & Young Children*, 19(3), 203–212.

Glaser, B. G. & Strauss, A. L. (1967). *Discovery of grounded theory: Strategies for qualitative research.* New York: Aldine.

Hamilton, R. & Bowers, B. J. (2005). Disclosing genetic test results to family members. *Journal of Nursing Scholarship*, 37(1), 18–24.

Hamilton, R. & Bowers, B. J. (In press). Convergence of age, genetic risk, and treatment decisions in young women (18–39y/o) at risk for hereditary breast and ovarian cancer. *Genetics in Medicine.*

Hughes, E. (1984). *The sociological eye: Selected papers* (rev. ed.). New Brunswick, NJ: Transaction Publishers.

Kools, S. (1997). Adolescent identity development in foster care. *Family Relations,* 46(3), 1–9.

Kools, S. (1999). Self-protection in adolescents in foster care. *Journal of Child and Adolescent Psychiatric Nursing*, 12(4), 139–152.

Kools, S. Gilliss, C. L., & Tong, E. M. (1999). Family transitions in congenital heart disease management: The impact of hospitalization in early adulthood. *Journal of Family Nursing*, 5(4), 427–448.

Kools, S. & Kennedy, C. (2002). Child sexual abuse treatment: Misinterpretation and mismanagement of child sexual behavior. *Child Care, Health and Development*, 28(3), 211–218.

Kools, S., McCarthy, M., Durham, R., & Robrecht, L. (1996). Dimensional analysis: Broadening the conception of grounded theory. *Qualitative Health Research*, 6(3), 312–330.

Kools, S. & Spiers, J. (2002). Caregiver understanding of adolescent development in residential treatment. *Journal of Child and Adolescent Psychiatric Nursing*, 15(4), 151–162.

Kools, S., Tong, E. M., Hughes, C. R., Jayne, R., Scheibly, K., Laughlin, J., & Gilliss, C. L. (2002). Hospital experiences of young adults with congenital heart disease: Divergence in expectations and dissonance in care. *American Journal of Critical Care*, 11(2), 115–127.

Liang, H. W. & Olshansky, E. (2005). The process of decision-making about care practices for children by caregivers who are Taiwanese temporary residents in the U.S.A. *The Journal of Pediatric Nursing*, 20(6), 453–460.

Lutz, B. & Bowers, B. J. (2005). The influence of disability on everyday life. *Qualitative Health Research*, 15(8), 1037–1054.

Lutz, B., Bowers, B. J., Esmond, S., & Jacobson, N. (2003). Improving primary care for persons with disabilities: The nature of expertise. *Disability & Society*, 18(4), 443–455.

McCarthy, M. (2003a). Situated clinical reasoning: Distinguishing acute confusion from dementia in hospitalized older adults. *Research in Nursing & Health*, 26(2), 90–101.

McCarthy, M.C. (2003b). Detecting acute confusion in older adults: Comparing clinical reasoning of nurses working in acute, long-term, and community health care environments. *Research in Nursing & Health*, 26(3), 203–212.

McCarthy, M., Ruiz, E., Gale, B., Moore, N., & Karem, C. (2004). The meaning of health: Perspectives of Anglo and Hispanic older women. *Health Care for Women International, Special Issue on Aging*, January.

Norton, S. & Bowers, B. J. (2001). Working toward consensus: Providers' strategies to shift patients from curative to palliative treatment choices. *Research in Nursing & Health*, 24(4), 258–269.

Olshansky, E. F. (1987a). Identity of self as infertile: An example of theory-generating research. *Advances in Nursing Science*, 9(2), 54–63.

Olshansky, E. F. (1987b). Infertility and its influence on women's career identities. *Health Care for Women International*, 8(2/3), 185–196.

Olshansky, E. F. (1993a). Application of dimensional analysis to qualitative research. (Moderator of session presented by Drs. L. Schatzman, A. Fisher, D. Hatton, N. Droes, E. Olshansky, M. McCarthy, & B. Bowers). *Communicating Nursing Research*, 26(1), 235–243.

Olshansky, E. F. (1993b). Application of dimensional analysis to a qualitative study of infertility. *Communicating Nursing Research*, 26(1), 241.

Olshansky, E. (2005). Feeling normal: Women's experiences of menopause after infertility. *MCN: The American Journal of Maternal Child Nursing*, 30(3), 195–200.

Pfeiffer, E. (1975). A short portable mental status questionnaire for the assessment of organic brain deficit in elderly patients. *Journal of the American Geriatrics Society*, 23, 433–441.

Schatzman, L. (1991). Dimensional analysis: Notes on an alternative approach to the grounding of theory in qualitative research. In D. Maines (Ed.), *Social organization and social process: Essays in honor of Anselm Strauss* (pp. 303–314). New York: Aldine de Gruyter.

Schatzman, L. & Strauss, A. L. (1973). *Field research: Strategies for a natural sociology*. Englewood Cliffs, NJ: Prentice-Hall, Inc.

Strauss, A. L. (1987). *Qualitative analysis for social scientists*. Cambridge: Cambridge University Press.

Strauss, A. L., Schatzman, L., Bucher, R., Ehrlich, D., & Sabshin, M. (1964). *Psychiatric ideologies and institutions*. London: The Free Press of Glencoe.

Watson, K. C., Kieckhefer, G. M., & Olshansky, E. (2006). Striving for therapeutic relationships: Parent-provider communication in the developmental treatment setting. *Qualitative Health Research*, 16(5), 647–663.

Example: Care-as-Service, Care-as-Relating, Care-as-Comfort

Understanding Nursing Home Residents' Definitions of Quality

Barbara Bowers, Barbara Fibich, and Nora Jacobson

The work of quality assurance (QA) has been described as encompassing three distinct tasks: defining quality, assessing quality, and assuring quality (Kane & Kane, 1988). Since the 1980s, health services researchers and policymakers have grown increasingly interested in incorporating the point of view of health care consumers into QA procedures (Davies & Ware, 1988). In the long-term care (LTC) arena, consumer perspectives have been used both to define the dimensions of quality (Grant, Reimer, & Bannatyne, 1996; Grau, Chandler, & Saunders, 1995; National Citizens' Coalition for Nursing Home Reform, 1985; Nores, 1997) and to prioritize the dimensions of quality that have been proposed by experts (Bliesmer & Earle, 1993; Mattiasson & Andersson, 1997; Pearson et al., 1993). The trend toward involving consumers in LTC QA has been codified in legislation: The Omnibus Budget Reconciliation Act of 1987 includes the requirement that quality measurements incorporate assessments of resident satisfaction.

In some conceptualizations of quality in health care, consumers can play a central role in assessing and defining quality. The approach known as "patient-centered" care uses patients' assessments of their quality of life to indicate the presence of high-quality care (Aller & Coeling, 1995; Gerteis et al., 1993; Lutz & Bowers, 2000; Mattiasson & Andersson, 1997; Miller, 1997; Pearson et al., 1993). A second approach views autonomy— manifested in active participation—as key to quality (Ashworth, Longmate, & Morrison, 1992; Jirovec & Maxwell, 1993; Kane et al., 1997;

Mitchell & Koch, 1997; Wetle et al., 1988). Here, individuals' perceptions of choice are used as one indicator of quality (Brocklehurst & Dickinson, 1996; Brooke & Short, 1996). A third approach conceptualizes quality care as care that meets the expectations of those who purchase it (Lengnick-Hall & Barton, 1995; Owens & Batchelor, 1996). Thus, quality is to be assessed through instruments that measure consumer satisfaction (Cleary & McNeil, 1988; Davis, Sebastian, & Tschetter, 1997; Jackson & Kroenke, 1997; Laitinen, 1994; Ludwig-Beymer et al., 1993; Pearson et al., 1993). A fourth approach uses ethnography to examine the experience—good or bad—of being a patient in the health care system or a resident in institutions devoted to restoring health or managing illness (Clark & Bowling, 1990; Goffman, 1961; Gubrium, 1975; Kane et al., 1997).

Although consumer perspectives are rarely the central determinant in overall assessments of quality, their use has provoked controversy. There is debate about how these views can best be gathered and used (Cleary & Edgman-Levitan, 1997; Lehr & Strosberg, 1991; Peters, 1993). Critics have argued that consumers cannot be competent judges of the technical elements of health care quality (Donabedian, 1980), seeing consumer quality assessments as more indicative of consumer characteristics and affective responses to interpersonal experiences than the actual quality of the service received (Grau et al., 1995; Larsson & Larsson, 1999). Defenders of the use of consumer quality assessment, however, citing studies that show good agreement between consumer assessments and a "gold standard" of expert assessment, assert that consumers *are* able to make competent judgments about the technical components of care (Davies & Ware, 1988). In addition, they argue that interpersonal experience constitutes an important dimension of quality, one that consumers are, in fact, uniquely qualified to assess (Carson, Carson, & Roe, 1998).

The characteristics of individuals who use LTC services have been seen as particularly problematic for including them in QA activities. Researchers have warned, for example, about threats to validity posed by factors like dementia, fatalistic resignation, low expectations, and fear of retaliation after unfavorable assessments (Aller & Coeling, 1995; Bliesmer & Earle, 1993; Grau et al., 1995; Laitinen, 1994; Pearson et al., 1993).

Despite these difficulties, several studies have sought to solicit the definitions of quality held by the residents of nursing homes. The most comprehensive—and the earliest—of these studies, a nationwide project conducted by the National Citizens' Coalition for Nursing Home Reform (1985), identified many of the dimensions of daily life in LTC facilities that were key to residents' ideas about quality of care. Overall, participants in this study defined quality care as having "choices and the ability to make them" (p. 15) in a happy, safe environment, being treated as individuals, and being allowed to be independent. Later studies have emphasized the importance of social relationships in residents' perceptions of quality care (Grant et al., 1996; Grau et al., 1995; Mattiasson & Andersson, 1997).

The current research was designed to expand on earlier work by looking at quality of care in an LTC facility from the residents' point of view. As this essay will show, residents' definitions of quality centered on the intricacies of their relationships with their care providers and on the consequences of care for physical comfort and sense of self.

Methods

The research for this project was part of a larger study that examined care and caregiving practices in several LTC facilities from multiple perspectives. The portion of the study reported here focused on how nursing home residents conceptualize the quality of their care. The researchers used in-depth interviews and grounded dimensional analysis (Caron & Bowers, 2000; Glaser & Strauss, 1967; Schatzman, 1991; Strauss, 1987) to collect and analyze the data.

Data were collected at three LTC facilities in and around Madison, Wisconsin. The facilities served a range of income levels and had minimal deficiencies as indicated by state survey results. To facilitate comparison to the wider market, these facilities were purposely selected to reflect different owner types, payment sources, and resident income levels. (For more information about the facilities, see Table 5.1.)

Following approval by the human subjects committee, residents were recruited into the study by facility nurses who provided no direct patient care. (Institutional Review Board approval was contingent on using a familiar staff person who was not a direct care provider to do the recruitment.) Researchers asked the nurses to invite participation from all residents who could understand what was being asked of them. The only residents nurses were instructed not to invite were those who were too ill or too cognitively impaired to participate in an interview. The nurses gave each resident a brief oral description of the research. Residents who were interested in participating completed a form indicating their name, room number, and a convenient time to contact them. The first nine residents in each facility to express an interest in participation were included in the research. (See Table 5.2 for more information about the residents.)

Early in the recruitment process, discussions between researchers and facility nurses revealed that the nurses were not recruiting residents they saw as "unrealistic" or "inappropriate" in their expectations. Further questioning revealed that these unchosen residents tended to be known to staff as "complainers" or as "difficult." Sensing that the perspective of complainers might provide interesting data about quality, the researchers asked nurses to include residents with this reputation in the study but not to reveal which residents were complainers until after all interviews were completed.

Interviews with residents took place in the residents' rooms, with only the resident and the interviewer present. Depending on the resident's stamina, interviews lasted between fifteen minutes and two hours; most lasted about forty-five minutes. Residents were initially asked only to "talk about what it's like to live here." The purpose of this request was to have residents identify for the researcher those elements of their daily lives that they themselves found most relevant. Residents rarely needed further prompting or encouragement to talk.

Resident responses to these general questions often resulted in an initial evaluative response such as "It's not so bad," "It's hell," "It's OK." Residents were then prompted to elaborate on these responses. In particular, they were asked to give examples of experiences they had had in the nursing home, to describe what they found either good or bad about these experiences, and to specify how they had come to these conclusions. Analysis of their responses to these probing questions sought to delineate the dimensions of both "good" and "bad" care as conceptualized by the residents. As the study progressed, second interviews were guided by emerging analysis to further elucidate the dimensions of the participants' experiences and perceptions of quality. All but one resident,

Table 5.1. *Characteristics of Long-Term Care Facilities*

	Facility 1	Facility 2	Facility 3
Facility type	For-profit	Not-for-profit	Not-for-profit
Facility management	National chain	Church-sponsored/ locally managed	Locally managed
Resident income level	Low to middle income	Middle and upper middle income	Upper income
Number of beds	103	184	64
Payment sources (by % residents)	70% Medicaid/9% Medicare/21% private pay	46% Medicaid/22% Medicare/32% private pay	100% private pay
Staffing levels	Above state-mandated minimums	Above state-mandated minimums	Above state-mandated minimums
Reputation in the community	Good	Good	Very good
State survey results	No level 3 deficiencies	No level 3 deficiencies	No level 3 deficiencies

who was discharged, were interviewed twice. The interval between interviews ranged from seven to ten days.

Interview data were analyzed using grounded dimensional analysis, an approach derived from grounded theory (Glaser & Strauss, 1967; Strauss, 1987) and dimensional analysis (Caron & Bowers, 2000; Schatzman, 1991). Grounded dimensional analysis combines the key elements

Table 5.2. *Characteristics of Participating Residents* (N = 26)

Facility representation	9 from Facility 1
	9 from Facility 2
	8 from Facility 3
Age range	64–104
Sex	21 women
	5 men
Lengths of stay	2 months–4 years
Functional status	14 independent (self-care; 7 or higher on SPMSQ* [Pfeiffer, 1975]); 12 dependent (requiring help with bathing, toileting, walking, dressing, eating; 6 or higher on SPMSQ)

*SMPSQ = Short Portable Mental Status Questionnaire.

of grounded theory, including theoretical sampling and constant comparison, with the analytic framework provided by dimensional analysis. This framework explicates the phenomenon of interest (care quality) by prompting the analyst to conduct a rigorous examination of the perspective from which the phenomenon is presented by the subjects, the context within which the phenomenon is described, the dimensions of the phenomenon, the conditions under which the phenomenon varies, and the consequences of the phenomenon.

In this study, analysis focused on how residents described the phenomenon of care, including identification of the dimensions of care or daily life that were used by residents when describing good or bad care. Comparative analyses across interviews suggested the three distinct types of resident quality definitions described in this chapter. Within each interview, there was a high level of consistency in the dimensions used to define quality. Further analysis of how these three types of definitions clustered by resident condition suggested that the definition of quality varied with level of functional impairment. Other variation in resident definitions of quality cannot be attributed easily to resident status. This variation and some of the implications are discussed below.

Results

Residents' descriptions of quality fell into three categories. These categories tended to cluster by the resident's level of dependency and by his or her reputation among nurses as "difficult." (The significance of these resident characteristics for their definitions of quality was identified during analysis; the researchers did not use functional status and reputation as a complainer as a priori categories in the design or execution of the study.) Among the more independent group of participants, residents identified by staff as complainers tended to see care-as-service, whereas residents identified as ranging from "more reasonable" to "real sweeties" usually described care-as-relating. The very dependent group of residents, however, some of whom were also identified by staff as complainers or manipulators, defined care-as-comfort.

Care-as-Service

There were four participants who described care-as-service. Two resided in Facility 2 and two in Facility 3—the homes that served a middle- and upper-income clientele. These residents used the term "service" to refer to the staff work—passing food trays, making beds, assisting with bathing and personal care—that providers and researchers generally label "care" or "caregiving." Residents who used the language of service focused on technical/instrumental aspects of care, including how well, how quickly, and how consistently the work was done. These residents perceived themselves as the purchasers of services and tended to compare their experiences in the LTC facilities with other instances in which they had paid people to provide them with specific services (e.g., appliance repair people or restaurant wait staff).

These residents suggested that they had the "rights" accruing to any consumer. For example, they believed that they should have the authority to instruct staff in how or when something should be done and that they were entitled to pass judgment on the adequacy of the services received: "When I'm paying so much I should have more to say. I'm paying good money to stay here, I should have better service. I pay $3,000 a month and I can't even get a glass of water when I want it."

Residents who conceptualized care as a purchased service made their own expectations important criteria for evaluating the quality of the care they were provided. As with other purchased services, their expectations for care had to do with value and work performed. These residents evaluated their care by how well the work was done, whether the outcome was of high quality, and whether the work was performed in a timely manner. They viewed themselves as active participants in evaluation, not simply the passive recipients of others' judgments of adequacy. They were often highly critical of the failure of their care providers to live up to their expectations and frustrated by their inability to perform formal evaluations of the staff. As one resident stated, "It isn't right but they just do it the way they want. I have nothing to say about it." Another resident used even stronger language: "It's like robbery .... you pay a fortune for a good place, thinking the service will be pretty good. Nobody has any pride in their work anymore. They just take your money and then you don't get the service you expect."

Residents who viewed care-as-service were likely to identify having to wait as particularly emblematic of poor quality service. When forced to wait, these residents made comments like: "I don't know why they don't train them better ... [they] can't even figure out the simplest things," "[They] have no understanding of what sick people really need," or "[They] are] so unorganized, I mean, [they] use 100 steps to do something that would take someone with more common sense only ten."

Other residents perceived waiting as a demonstration of an implicit social hierarchy, and aides' wish to keep them at the bottom. These residents saw waiting as part of a power struggle, attributing specific motives to the care providers who made them wait: "It's not that they're so busy you know ... sometimes they're just standing around they want to make sure we know our place ... [and] know who's in charge" or "They do it on purpose, you know ... [making us wait] gives them a feeling of power."

Some residents who grew impatient with waiting described taking matters into their own hands, at times placing themselves in some physical jeopardy. In an effort to call attention to the unresponsiveness of some care providers, they were likely to make their actions, and the risks they had taken, widely known to the supervisory staff. According to these residents, this kind of "complaining" angered their care providers, but was effective in prompting at least a temporary increase in staff responsiveness.

Care-as-Relating

Sixteen participants—six in Facility 1, three in Facility 2, and seven in Facility 3—defined care-as-relating. When asked about care quality, these residents spoke about their relationships with staff. They emphasized the degree of closeness they experienced in these relationships, rarely mentioning actual caregiving activities or tasks. When pressed to speak specifically about the care they received, care-as-relating residents talked almost exclusively about the affect of their caregivers, their caregivers' motivation, and the evidence of real friendship that they found in their relationships.

Good care was described as care that was given by someone who "really likes her work ... really cares about the people here." Care-as-relating residents spoke less about the technical aspects of care (the how and when described by care-as-service residents), but more about the signs of individualized affection and friendship they found in the care they received. Even under direct questioning about the technical aspects of care, these residents refused to acknowledge that it had any importance to them, insisting that factors such as competence were irrelevant. For example, residents were consistently willing to overlook care that might lead to poor outcomes if the caregiver's intent was consistent with a caring relationship. The woman quoted here, for example, excused an aide's failure to assist her with her daily exercises, including ambulation: "It's OK ... you know really. ... It doesn't matter so much. ... I'll get along. ... She's so sweet and tries so hard ... and I wouldn't want to hurt her feelings."

Care-as-relating residents identified aides' willingness to share information about their personal lives, especially personal troubles, as an example of high-quality care. One resident described a favored aide: "She's really sweet, a good listener. She tells me about problems with her husband ... and I give her advice." As suggested by this quote, care-as-relating residents saw reciprocity as evidence of good relationships, and thus of good quality care. Residents often discussed reciprocity in terms of sharing invisible or past personal identities. An aide would share with the resident previously unknown personal details related to her life outside of work; in turn, the resident could share personal identities from his or her past. "Good" aides were described as attending to these identities as they provided care. By so doing, these aides were acknowledging resident selves other than those related to old age, illness, and disability. As one resident noted, a good aide was one who could "see me as not just an old lady or someone with bad knees and a catheter to clean."

By contrast, "bad" care was described as care that was given by someone who had "a bad attitude," who "obviously doesn't like her job," who "never smiles or looks me in the eye," who "doesn't keep promises," who "treats me like I'm invisible or stupid," or who "never just chats, you know ... [is] just all business." Bad care was conceptualized by care-as-relating residents as care given by a provider who seemed to strive to minimize or eliminate the interactive dimensions of care and whose motivation was mercenary, rather than affective (i.e., aides who were "just in it for the money," rather than out of a desire to help people).

Although residents who described care-as-relating were as likely as those who described care-as-service to experience waiting, the meaning they attributed to waiting and their response to waiting provide a sharp contrast to care-as-service residents. They did not see having to wait as demonstrating poor quality care. Rather, care-as-relating residents tended to excuse long waits in ways that suggested they were determined to absolve their caregivers of any responsibility for making them wait. Their comments about having to wait included: "[It's] no one's fault, really ... just too much work to do" or "The girls work so hard, you know ...

[they're] so overworked and short-staffed … they get there as quick as they can."

Like care-as-service residents, care-as-relating residents sometimes described reacting to waiting by taking matters into their own hands. What they intended by doing so, however, was quite different. These residents saw taking action as an opportunity for them to demonstrate reciprocity. They described doing things for themselves to "save the girls time." As one woman said, "They do so much and work so hard. I try to find little ways to take some of the burden off." Some accounts suggested that these acts of reciprocity could endanger the resident. For example, a resident might mention to an aide that she had climbed over her bed rails so that she would not have to "bother" the aide with a request for her to lower them. Residents continued to take such risks, even when the intended recipient had objected: "She always scolds me but I know she really appreciates it. It's our secret." In keeping the action a "secret" between resident and caregiver, care-as-relating residents were demonstrating that they saw their actions as a means to strengthen interpersonal relationships, and not as ways to manipulate staff into providing better service.

Being able to reciprocate in this way was viewed as rewarding, particularly for residents who saw themselves as kind and helpful and unlikely to make "unreasonable" demands or to expect to be "waited on" by others. The following comment was typical: "I've always prided myself in helping out where I can. I'm the sort of person who doesn't ask unless I really have to." "Helping out" allowed residents to assert a treasured self: that of the uncomplaining, thoughtful friend.

Care-as-Comfort

Frailer, more dependent residents tended to describe quality as care that was directed at maintaining their physical comfort. Six participants—three each at Facilities 1 and 2 (the low- and moderate-income facilities)—defined care-as-comfort. Unlike the less frail residents who focused on care-as-service and care-as-relating, these residents expressed tremendous concern about the specific hands-on care provided by aides. Although this group, like the care-as-relating residents, also mentioned the importance of having good relationships with staff, they viewed good relationships primarily as the means to ensure that they would receive timely assistance from aides.

The assistance that these residents found to be the most important was related to physical comfort, rather than to medical treatment, safety, or the routine mandated tasks that aides do for residents (i.e., bed making, bathing, cleaning the rooms). Residents' accounts of good quality care were frequently focused on having something "just right." Maintaining a sense of "just right" required attending to very small, often invisible, increments of bodily changes that were generally not appreciated by staff. For example, these residents described how propping up an aching leg in just the right position could make a huge difference between comfort and "terrible" discomfort. Similarly, the difference between a refreshing drink of water and one that was offensive was, literally, a matter of degree. The discrepancy between the apparent magnitude of these differences as perceived by staff and the significance for the residents was huge.

Residents who sensed the staff's resentment grew frustrated and angry, both with the staff and with themselves:

I tell them I have to go to the bathroom and I can't wait and they still don't come. It's cruel to make someone wait when they know it'll mean an accident. Sometimes I can't go and they get so disgusted, and even if they don't, I feel bad. I'm taking up their time.

As suggested by this quote, loss of the ability to read body cues (a loss related to age and, often, the side effects of numerous medications and treatments) exacerbated the repetitive and sometimes unproductive nature of the tasks that residents required for their personal comfort. Staff did come to resent repeated requests to do these tasks and often began to contest residents' attempts to read their own body cues: "No, you don't have to go to the bathroom, we just took you and you didn't have to go, remember?" or "You couldn't possibly be cold, it's 82 degrees in here."

The uncertainty attached to reading body cues created a dilemma for residents: to ask for assistance or not to ask? The consequences of making the wrong decision, in either direction, were significant. Residents who suspected that they had to urinate, but weren't sure, for example, ran the risk either of wetting the bed, an event that created further discomfort, humiliation, resentment, and, eventually, more work for the staff, or of antagonizing their caregivers by asking for help with what might turn out to be an "unnecessary" trip to the toilet. Because they wished to minimize unnecessary work and didn't want to gain reputations for "crying wolf," residents often selected "waiting until I can't stand it" as the most reasonable, albeit agonizing, option.

Discussion

The three conceptualizations of quality described by the nursing home residents who participated in this study show some areas of overlap with those specified in the definitions of quality proffered by experts: The care-as-service residents, for example, fit well into the consumerist model of those who seek to assess quality by measuring consumer satisfaction. The wide range in resident-derived definitions of quality, however points out the inadequacy of relying on one conceptualization of quality for QA procedures. For example, consumer satisfaction surveys that focus on the technical aspects of care might be rejected by care-as-relating residents because these residents view themselves as friends, not consumers, and would see criticizing their caregivers as disloyal. Instruments to measure choice would be perceived as ironic, at the least, and even as cruel by the care-as-comfort residents for whom "autonomy" means choosing to suffer rather than antagonize their caregivers. Care-as-service residents would likely reject the idea that facilities have any right to determine the dimensions that compose their "quality of life," but would see such attempts as presumptuous, not the place of those whose purpose is to serve. However, this group may well be the most credible source of consumer satisfaction assessment because they are willing to provide negative judgments.

The significance of these findings lies primarily in their implications for the measurement of care quality and for how knowledge about quality can be applied to practice. First, the current emphasis on expert-defined clinical aspects of care, such as those encompassed by the minimum data set quality indicators (MDS/QI), does not acknowledge the complexity of quality as experienced by nursing home residents. From the point of view of most residents, focusing regulation and practice efforts solely on improving or maintaining these clinical dimensions may not result in adequate quality of care as they themselves define it. The findings reported here provide support for the current Health Care Financing Administration–funded efforts to develop an MDS specifically directed at resident quality of life. For example, care-as-relating would fit more easily into quality of life than it does into the domains that measure quality of care. Care-as-service and care-as-comfort, however, cannot be neatly placed into either category. In particular, comfort, as described by the residents who participated in this research, is not captured by either quality of care or quality of life. The closest category currently found in the MDS is pain. This category is, however, practically and conceptually different from what residents described. Addition of a new "comfort domain" might improve the ability of the MDS to assess quality in a way that is meaningful to residents.

These findings also have important implications for two areas of practice: determining the staffing needs required to deliver quality care and improving clinical practice. Currently, there are no federally mandated staffing rules for nursing homes except the requirement that staffing be adequate to ensure high-quality care. The staffing levels necessary to provide such care, however, are highly contested (Bowers, Esmond, & Jacobson, 2000). Most attempts to determine "adequate" staffing levels base their assessments on associations between staffing and results on the MDS/QI. As this study has suggested, these expert-defined clinical dimensions may not capture what constitutes quality for nursing home residents. As applied to clinical practice, these findings have significant implications for resident needs assessment, care planning, in-service education, and staff supervision. An understanding of the resident definitions described in this essay would improve practitioners' ability to plan and deliver individualized care and to evaluate the quality of care provided in ways that are meaningful to residents.

The limitations of the work reported here are largely inherent to the exploratory nature of the study and to the interpretive methodology used. The small sample size allowed greater analytic richness but was inadequate to ensure external validity. The study was cross-sectional. Researchers were unable to ascertain if residents' conceptualizations of quality shift over time. For example, as suggested by one of the anonymous reviewers of this essay, it may be that residents become increasingly "institutionalized" as their stays lengthen, adopting definitions of quality that are more congruent with those of their care providers. The design of this study also did not allow linkages between resident conceptualizations of quality and resident characteristics such as socioeconomic (SES) or functional status.

In the future, it will be important to determine the generalizability of the three types of care quality definitions described here. Further research might test the associations between functional status (and characteristics like SES, race, and gender) and resident definitions of care quality. It might also develop a "natural history" of resident conceptualizations of quality through longitudinal study and look at the relationship between resident perceptions of quality and contextual factors such as facility staffing levels and the nature of resident/staff relationships.

References

Aller, L. J. & Coeling, H. V. (1995). Quality of life: Its meaning to the long-term care resident. *Journal of Gerontological Nursing*, 21(2), 20–25.

Ashworth, P. D., Longmate, M. A., & Morrison, P. (1992). Patient participation: Its meaning and significance in the context of caring. *Journal of Advanced Nursing*, 17(12), 1430–1439.

Bliesmer, M. & Earle, P. (1993). Nursing home quality perceptions. *Journal of Gerontological Nursing*, 19(6), 27–34.

Bowers, B. J., Esmond, S., & Jacobson, N. (2000). The relationship between staffing and quality in long term care facilities: Exploring the views of nurse aides. *Journal of Nursing Care Quality*, 14(4), 55–64.

Brocklehurst, J. & Dickinson, E. (1996). Autonomy for elderly people in long-term care. *Age and Ageing*, 25(4), 329–332.

Brooke, V. M. & Short, R. A. (1996). Measuring the perception of choices in the nursing home. *Journal of Nursing Measurement*, 4(2), 103–115.

Caron, C. D. & Bowers, B. J. (2000). Methods and application of dimensional analysis: A contribution to concept and knowledge development in nursing. In B. L. Rodgers & K. A. Knafl (Eds.), *Concept development in nursing: Foundations, techniques, and applications*, 2nd ed. (pp. 285–320). Philadelphia: Saunders.

Carson, P. P., Carson, K. D., & Roe, C. W. (1998). Toward understanding the patient's perception of quality. *Health Care Supervisor*, 16(3), 36–42.

Clark, P. & Bowling, A. (1990). Quality of everyday life in long stay institutions for the elderly. An observational study of long stay hospital and nursing home care. *Social Science and Medicine*, 30(11), 1201–1210.

Cleary, P. D. & Edgman-Levitan, S. (1997). Health care quality: Incorporating consumer perspectives. *Journal of the American Medical Association*, 278(19), 1608–1612.

Cleary, P. D. & McNeil, B. J. (1988). Patient satisfaction as an indicator of quality care. *Inquiry*, 25(1), 25–36.

Davies, A. R. & Ware, J. E. (1988). Involving consumers in quality of care assessment. *Health Affairs*, 7(1), 33–48.

Davis, M. A., Sebastian, J. G., & Tschetter, J. (1997). Measuring quality of nursing home service: Residents' perspective. *Psychological Reports*, 81(2), 531–542.

Donabedian, A. (1980). *Exploration in quality assessment and monitoring: The definitions of quality and approaches to its assessment.* Ann Arbor, MI: Health Administration Press.

Gerteis, M., Edgman-Levitan, S., Daley, J., & Delbanco, T. L. (Eds.). (1993). *Through the patient's eyes: Understanding and promoting patient-centered care.* San Francisco: Jossey-Bass.

Glaser, B. G. & Strauss, A. L. (1967). *The discovery of grounded theory.* Chicago: Aldine.

Goffman, E. (1961). *Asylums.* Garden City, NY: Anchor Books.

Grant, N. K., Reimer, M., & Bannaryne, J. (1996). Indicators of quality in long-term care facilities. *International Journal of Nursing Studies,* 33(5), 469–478.

Grau, L., Chandler, B., & Saunders, C. (1995). Nursing home residents' perceptions of the quality of their care. *Journal of Psychosocial Nursing,* 33(5), 34–41.

Gubrium, J. F. (1975). *Living and dying at Murray Manor.* New York: St. Martin's Press.

Jackson, J. L. & Kroenke, K. (1997). Patient satisfaction and quality of care. *Military Medicine,* 162(4), 273–277.

Jirovec, M. M. & Maxwell, B. A. (1993). Nursing home residents' functional ability and perceptions of choice. *Journal of Gerontological Nursing,* 19(9), 10–14.

Kane, R. A., Caplan, A. L., Urv-Wong, E. K., Freeman, I. C., Aroskar, M. A., & Finch, M. (1997). Everyday matters in the lives of nursing home residents: Wish for and perception of choice and control. *Journal of the American Geriatrics Society,* 45(9), 1086–1093.

Kane, R. A., & Kane, R. L. (1988). Long-term care: Variations on a quality assurance theme. *Inquiry,* 25(1), 132–146.

Laitinen, P. (1994). Elderly patients' and their informal caregivers' perception of care given: The study-control ward design. *Journal of Advanced Nursing,* 20(1), 71–76.

Larsson, B. W. & Larsson, G. (1999). Patients' views on quality of care: Do they merely reflect their sense of coherence? *Journal of Advanced Nursing,* 30(1), 33–39.

Lehr, H. & Strosberg, M. (1991). Quality improvement in health care: Is the patient still left out? *Quarterly Research Bulletin,* 17, 326–329.

Lengnick-Hall, C. A. & Barton, W. F. (1995). The patient as pivot point for quality in health care delivery. *Hospital & Health Services Administration,* 40(1), 25–39.

Ludwig-Beymer, P., Ryan, C. J., Johnson, N. J., Hennessy, K. A., Gattuso, M. C., Epsom, R., & Czurylo, K. (1993). Using patient perceptions to improve quality care. *Journal of Nursing Care Quality,* 7(2), 42–51.

Lutz, B. J. & Bowers, B. J. (2000). Patient-centered care: Understanding its interpretation and implementation in health care. *Scholarly Inquiry for Nursing Practice: An International Journal,* 14(2), 165–182.

Mattiasson, A-C. & Andersson, L. (1997). Quality of nursing home care assessed by competent nursing home patients. *Journal of Advanced Nursing*, 26(6), 1117–1124.

Miller, N. A. (1997). Patient-centered long-term care. *Health Care Financing Review*, 19(2), 1–10.

Mitchell, P. & Koch, T. (1997). An attempt to give nursing home residents a voice in the quality improvement process: The challenge of frailty. *Journal of Clinical Nursing*, 6(6), 453–461.

National Citizens' Coalition for Nursing Home Reform. (1985). *A consumer perspective on quality care: The residents' point of view*. Washington, DC: Author.

Nores, T. H. (1997). What is most important for elders in institutional care in Finland? *Geriatric Nursing*, 18(2), 67–69.

Owens, D. J. & Batchelor, C. (1996). Patient satisfaction and the elderly. *Social Science and Medicine*, 42(11), 1483–1491.

Pearson, A., Hocking, S., Mort, S., & Riggs, A. (1993). Quality of care in nursing homes: From the resident's perspective. *Journal of Advanced Nursing*, 18(1), 20–24.

Peters, D. A. (1993). Improving quality requires consumer input: Using focus groups. *Journal of Nursing Care Quality*, 7(2), 34–41.

Schatzman, L. (1991). Dimensional analysis: Notes on an alternative approach to the grounding of theory in qualitative research. In D. R. Maines (Ed.), *Social organization and social process* (pp. 303–314). New York: Aldine De Gruyter.

Strauss, A. L. (1987). *Qualitative analysis for social scientists*. Cambridge: Cambridge University Press.

Wetle, T., Levkoff, S., Cwikel, J., & Rosen, A. (1988). Nursing home resident participation in medical decisions: Perceptions and preferences. *The Gerontologist*, 28(Suppl.), 32–38.

Dialogue: Questions?

Q: What I think about as theoretical sensitivity is the lens that I bring to the research—and that's not language or meaning that I've heard much of today, and I guess I just want to ask you if you'd comment on that?

Barbara: Yes, sure. Well I guess in thinking about theoretical sensitivity. I was reading Anselm's 1987 book again recently, and there was a place in there where he gives a demonstration of what he calls theoretical sensitivitsm, which Lennie [Schatzman] would call "recognition recall." It was a set of concepts that he clearly already had used—I think of it as a "pet concept." I guess my understanding of theoretical sensitivity is different than this. I think of it as *the ability to render something abstract or conceptual, to move to a more theoretical level.* This is quite different than the ability to find a theory or theoretical concept to use to explain something. They are of course, both important conceptual activities, recognition-recall and theoretical sensitivity, but not the same things.

Q: I'm trying to cognitize the whole notion of dimensional analysis. You refer at one point to researchers developing distance between themselves and the problem, and I was wondering *how* a person goes about creating that distance?

Barbara: Maybe I wasn't very clear. It is *not* the goal of a researcher to create distance between them self and the phenomenon. The point is actually to minimize the distance. However, when you start engaging in comparative analysis very early in analysis you are bringing things from your own experience, or those of the research team—your discipline, from what you read last Saturday—to conjure those comparisons that you use. And as soon as you do that, you are using sources external to your data to create those comparisons. That, in fact, distances you from your data. So, don't do that early; wait until later, until you have grounded yourself in the data you have. The more you have generated from your data before you engage in comparisons with things outside your data, the more grounded you are likely to be.

So what you should do is to listen carefully to the dimensions that are called out by the informants, or the research participants, and use those as your bank of dimensions to work with for your analysis, rather than what you bring from your own experiences, because what you bring is distancing.

Q: If that's the reason you distance yourself, another algorithm for measuring distance from that point may be a dimensional algorithm. What are the steps or procedures to try and do that?

Barbara: Well I probably wouldn't try to measure it. But I don't know how you'd trace this—by that I mean, you couldn't see the process by looking at the finished product. It's a matter of using your memos and tracing your decisions along the way to see if your comparisons and the structures that you start to create in your coding system come from the interviews, that you were not directive early in the study. I mean, I'm certainly very directive in later interviews. So, if you do very little directing in the beginning and then use the dimensions that informants identify, rather than ones you bring, that is less distancing!

6. Shifting the Grounds
Constructivist Grounded Theory Methods

Kathy Charmaz

By its fortieth anniversary year, grounded theory had become an acclaimed method in diverse fields. Scholars treat several of its strategies as standard practice in qualitative inquiry and as part of the general lexicon in qualitative research. Researchers have widely adopted coding and memo-writing strategies, although they may use them in somewhat different ways than grounded theorists do. And, of course, as grounded theorists, we differ among ourselves on which strategies we adopt and how we use them.

Grounded theorists who use some version of the method share much in common—but differ on several foundational assumptions that shape our studies. (I leave out all those who merely claim grounded theory to legitimize conducting inductive qualitative research.) Grounded theory methods provide a frame for qualitative inquiry and guidelines for conducting it. We may have different starting points and conceptual agendas, yet we all begin with inductive logic, subject our data to rigorous analysis, aim to develop theoretical analyses, and value grounded theory studies for informing policy and practice. All variants of grounded theory offer helpful strategies for collecting, managing, and analyzing qualitative data.

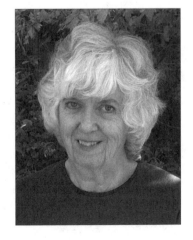

Anselm Strauss and Juliet Corbin (1994) observe that grounded theory has become a general method. They define a general method as having two major characteristics: (1) It is applicable in studies in diverse substantive areas and disciplines and (2) it provides a way to think about and conceptualize data, which may include inventing new analytic procedures. Strauss and Corbin imply that the mode of interrogating data remains consistent across studies in widely ranging substantive areas. My view of grounded theory as a general method, however, broadens the scope of its generality because our various grounded theory allegiances have spawned differences in how we think about and act toward data. I see grounded theory as an umbrella covering several different variants, emphases, and directions—and ways to think about data. In short, grounded theory represents a constellation of methods that we illuminate in our chapters in this book (see also Bryant & Charmaz, 2007b). As Karen Henwood (Charmaz & Henwood, 2008; Henwood & Pidgeon, 2003) has pointed out, we can see grounded theory not as a unitary method but as a useful nodal point around which researchers discuss contemporary debates in qualitative inquiry—and I believe, by extension, the production of knowledge and scientific theorizing.

In *The Discovery of Grounded Theory*,[1] Barney G. Glaser and Anselm L. Strauss (1967) set forth a powerful rhetoric of change from the quantitative canon to legitimize qualitative inquiry. They offered explicit strategies and inspired generations of graduate students, most of whom read no further and had scant knowledge of how to put grounded theory strategies into practice.[2] These students' limited understanding of grounded theory contributed to spreading diffuse understandings of the method later and, by default, to making grounded theory a general method, rather than a unitary one.[3]

But perhaps most significantly, Glaser and Strauss brought together their two contrasting philosophical and methodological traditions: Columbia University positivism and University of Chicago pragmatism, respectively. The positivist tradition emphasizes "*the* scientific method" and assumes an external world about which an unbiased observer can discover abstract generalities that explain empirical phenomena. Facts and values are separate in the positivist tradition. In contrast, the pragmatist tradition views reality as consisting of fluid, somewhat indeterminate processes. Pragmatism also acknowledges multiple perspectives emerging from people's actions to solve problems in their worlds (Charmaz, 2006; Mead 1934). Facts and values are joined in the pragmatist tradition. Although both positivists and pragmatists see truth as conditional and subject to revision, they have different starting points, modes of thought, and emphases in research practice.

When the collaboration of Glaser and Strauss began, Glaser (1991) had just embarked on his career. They focused on conceptualizing data from their project on the social organization of dying. Among many other lessons that Glaser recounts learning from collaborating with Strauss was "learning to deal constructively with [their] differences in thought and theory" (Glaser, 1991, p. 11).[4] Yet these differences were consequential. The union of Glaser and Strauss's rather disparate traditions placed grounded theory on somewhat unsteady ontological and epistemological grounds and planted the seeds of divergent directions for the method.

In this chapter, I take up the implications of ontological and epistemological divergence among grounded theorists and re-view the current directions of the method in light of changes during the last forty years. My approach to grounded theory preserves useful strategies that Glaser (Glaser, 1978; Glaser & Strauss, 1967) articulated. In fact, it preserves a strategy or two that he created but has discarded. It also preserves the pragmatist underpinnings of grounded theory but turns them back on the research process rather than only outward to the empirical world. Turning back and examining ourselves, our research situations, and our research process and products is consequential. We can learn to recognize our standpoints, adopt new perspectives, and turn in different directions than colleagues who focus exclusively on their research participants. Turning back prompts us to examine how *we* construct and reconstruct reality.

Shifting Ontological and Epistemological Grounds

Defining Constructivist Grounded Theory

The ontological and epistemological grounds of the grounded theory method have shifted in forty years, most recently with the constructivist challenge. What does constructivist grounded theory mean? How does it challenge prior grounded theory conceptions and practices? In brief, constructivist grounded theory is a contemporary revision of Glaser and Strauss's (1967; Glaser, 1978) classic grounded theory. It assumes a relativist epistemology, sees knowledge as socially produced, acknowledges multiple standpoints of both the research participants and the grounded theorist, and takes a reflexive stance toward our actions, situations, and participants in the field setting—and our analytic constructions of them

(Charmaz, 2000, 2006, 2007a, 2008a, 2008b). As Adele Clarke (2003, 2005, 2006, 2007) argues eloquently, the research reality is a situation that includes who and what is in that situation or affects it from the outside. A real world exists but is never separate from the viewer who may see it from multiple standpoints and whose views may conflict with research participants' standpoints and realities. Of course, our research participants' actions may also reveal sharp differences among themselves.

Constructivist grounded theory assumes that we produce knowledge by grappling with empirical problems. Knowledge rests on social constructions. We construct research processes and products, but these constructions occur under preexisting structural conditions, arise in emergent situations, and are influenced by the researcher's perspectives, privileges, positions, interactions, and geographical locations. All these conditions inhere in the research situation but in most studies remain unmentioned or are completely ignored.[5] Which observations we make, how we make them, and the views that we form of them reflect these conditions as do our subsequent grounded theories. Constructivists realize that conducting and writing research are not neutral acts. Unlike most authors, Monica J. Casper (1998) describes her study of the making of the unborn patient as "unashamedly politically engaged" (p. 25) because from the beginning she defined her topic as intertwined with reproductive health and abortion politics. She realized that fetal surgery posed risks to both the mother and the fetus and saw that the surgeons viewed the mother as a container for the fetus, the "real" patient, a stance with which she disagreed. Casper makes her starting points and perspectives explicit in the following statement:

> I have spent a great deal of time and energy articulating the ways in which fetal surgery and its practitioners are political. Yet I have also had to be reflexive about my own politics and how they have shaped this research. As C. Wright Mills argued, "there is no way in which any social scientist can avoid assuming choices of value and implying them in his [sic] work as a whole. ... No one is 'outside society'; the question is where each stands within it.".... My deep commitment to women's health issues and my reproductive rights philosophy generated my initial interest in fetal surgery. After beginning this project, I realized that moving from "activist" to "analyst" was not a simple endeavor; I could not just "turn off" my politics once I entered the field. To assert that I could somehow manage to keep my

politics separate from my research, while simultaneously exposing my informants' politics, would have been the height of methodological hypocrisy. (1997, pp. 240–241)

Constructivists enter participants' liminal world of meaning and action in ways classic grounded theorists do not. We aim to get as close to the empirical realities as possible. Constructivists favor thorough knowledge over efficient completion of our analyses. From a constructivist view, what we see, when, how, and to what extent we see it are not straightforward. Much remains tacit; much remains silent. We exist in a world that is acted upon and interpreted—by our research participants and by us—as well as being affected by other people and circumstances. Yet actions, interpretations, and influences may be unstated or go unrecognized. Our task is to make them explicit in our analyses. We interpret our research participants' actions and interpretations and try to locate their situations in the relevant circumstances. We try to get it right in the sense of trying to understand our research participants' beliefs, their purposes, the actions they take, and reasons for their actions and inactions from their perspectives.

We also try to locate participants' meanings and actions in larger social structures and discourses of which they may be unaware. Participants' meanings may reflect ideologies; their actions may reproduce current social conventions or power relationships. We look for the assumptions on which participants construct their meanings and actions. Assumptions of individual responsibility for health, for example, often lie beneath how people account for becoming ill, including their own as well as other individuals' illnesses. Holding such assumptions quickly leads to blame and to further beliefs that individuals can—and should—ameliorate their problems. Hence, social causes and solutions remain invisible. By locating our participants' meanings and actions in this way, we show the connections between micro and macro levels of analysis and thus link the subjective and the social.

As we constructivists develop our analyses, we know full well that we offer an interpretation contingent on our knowledge of our participants and their situations. Constructivists view data as constructed rather than discovered, and we see our analyses as interpretive renderings not as objective reports or the only viewpoint on the topic. As a result, we increase our awareness of the relativity not only in the empirical world with its multiple realities but also of our analyses. Such awareness fosters taking a reflexive stance throughout the research and writing processes. Casper's description of her research indicates the depth of her involvement and the travails of reflexive inquiry: "I have been moved and transformed by this research in multiple ways, and fetal surgery is something I shall continue to think and talk about long after this book is published. My politics and intellectual assumptions have been shaken time and again" (1998, p. 25).

In these two short sentences, Casper shows us that our research can prompt reflexivity throughout the process, *if* we plunge in and attempt to seek and understand the multiple perspectives of multiple participants, including our own. She recognized that treating fetal surgery as a women's health issue meant acknowledging that women chose the procedure as well as portraying enormous—and risky—consequences it could create for them. From the beginning, Casper's views of the implications of fetal surgery for women's reproductive health clashed with those of fetal surgeons whose views and work formed a significant part of her research. Unlike the experience of most qualitative researchers, Casper's early analytic work became known to those she criticized. After sharing a paper with one woman she had interviewed, the woman sent it to her surgical team. These surgeons confronted Casper about her beliefs and actions in the field and forced her to take a reflexive stance. What made Casper's study such a powerful analysis is exactly what made it so difficult. She immersed herself in studying a contested problem controlled by elites and did so as a young female graduate student.[6]

More commonly, qualitative researchers choose ordinary problems of ordinary folk. A reflexive stance may become apparent when researchers study an experience that they themselves share. David Karp (1996) wrote an insightful analysis in his study of people with depression, *Speaking of Sadness: Depression, Disconnection, and the Meanings of Illness*. He gives the reader clues that he has experienced depression when he suggests the position from which he writes in the first sentence of his acknowledgments.

> Most authors find it difficult to distance themselves from their writing. Issues, worked on nearly daily for years, become so familiar that bringing them into clear focus sometimes seems impossible. Problems of perspective are further compounded, when, as in this case, books are motivated by features of authors' lives that are at the core of their identities. (p. v)

Karp constructs the backdrop for his book in the opening sentence of his first chapter:

In a greater or lesser degree I have grappled with depression for almost 20 years. I suppose that even as a child my experience of life was as much characterized by anxiety as by joy and pleasure. And as I look back, there were lots of tip-offs that things weren't right. I find it difficult to remember much of my early years, but throughout high school and college I felt uncertain of myself, feared that I could not accomplish what was expected of me and had plenty of sleepless nights. At college one of my room-mates nicknamed me "weak heart," after a character-type in Dostoyevsky novels because I often seemed a bit of a lost soul. During all those years, though, I had no real baseline for evaluating the "normalcy" of my feelings. … It wasn't until my early thirties that I was forced to conclude that something was "really wrong" with me. (p. 3)

Karp's disclosures create a tone of authenticity for his subsequent analysis. In a sense, he casts himself as a double expert—an insider who has lived the studied experience and the social scientist who analyzes it. The images of himself as a boy who was different elicit readers' empathy and desire to learn more of his story. Throughout the book, Karp reflects on his own experience as he crafts an analysis of his interviews with people who have experienced depression. Karp's book is compelling because his personal stories foreshadow central points in his analysis but do not overshadow the empirical richness of his data or the analytic impact of the sociological narrative.

In the two narratives above, both authors wrote telling reflexive statements about their studies. Other scholars may take a deeply reflexive stance throughout their work without making public disclosures. Silences, too, may arise from considered decisions and reflect ethical choices about the research process, participants, and /or significant concerns about privacy.

Shifting Views of Grounded Theory

Why *constructivist* grounded theory? I refer to my position as constructivist for two main reasons. First, I seek to take reflexivity into explicit and continuous account. Second, I intend to distinguish it from earlier forms of social constructionism that viewed the research participants' actions as constructed but not their researchers' actions or situations. My form of constructivism, however, does not subscribe to the radical subjectivism and individual reductionism assumed by some advocates of constructivism. In such analyses, individual consciousness explains all. Social locations, cultural traditions, and interactional and situational contingencies are unrecognized. In contrast, constructivist grounded theory aims to position the research relative to the social circumstances impinging on it.

Other questions arise about grounded theory and by extension, its constructivist revision. Is grounded theory solely an interview method? My notion of grounded theory invokes a basic disciplinary assumption in sociology: Our data collection methods flow *from* the research question (Charmaz, 2006). Thus, a particular data collection or analytic strategy cannot drive the research question. This principle brings methodological eclecticism into grounded theory and counters those scholars who have treated it as a method for interview studies—only. Methodological eclecticism negates views of grounded theory and ethnography as mutually exclusive approaches and rejects views asserting the incompatibility of grounded theory with documents. Clearly, successively shaping and controlling the data works best, but documents may be all the data that researchers can obtain. Grounded theorists who have studied the history of science have excelled in using documents as their major source of data (see, for example, Bowker & Star, 1999; Clarke, 1998; Star, 1989; Star & Griesemer, 1989).

Does grounded theory necessitate adopting a symbolic interactionist perspective? No again. Similar to my view of data collection methods, I contend that grounded theorists can invoke diverse theoretical starting points to *open* inquiry such as feminist theory, poststructuralism, Marxist theory, or symbolic interactionism (Charmaz, 1990, 2005). I agree with Clarke (2005, 2006) that symbolic interactionism and grounded theory make a powerful "theory-methods package" (Fujimura, 1992; Star, 1989), although grounded theory strategies may be used from other theoretical starting points as well. Moreover, few grounded theorists subscribe to a symbolic interactionist theoretical orthodoxy—or any other kind of orthodoxy. Many of us draw on a range of concepts and theories as part of the analytic repertoire that we use with symbolic interactionism.

If grounded theorists have much in common, why is grounded theory a contested method? Various proponents have argued about what grounded theory is, whose version is correct, and what direction the method should take. The notion of a constellation of grounded theory methods has been recent and is symbolized by the production of *The Handbook of Grounded Theory*. Nonetheless, scholars within grounded theory (Charmaz, 2000, 2006; Clarke, 2005; Corbin, 1998; Glaser, 1992, 2002; Locke, 1996) and without it (Atkinson, Coffey, & Delamont, 2003; Burawoy, 1991; Cisnero-Puebla, 2007; Layder, 1998) have treated grounded theory as a contested method. Criticisms of grounded theory or a particular variant of it range from those of scholars who appear to have read nothing about grounded theory since 1967 to those who attend closely to discussions of the method.[7]

The originators' differences about which grounded theory strategies to adopt, what they entail, and how to put them into practice have elicited considerable discussion among their followers and commentators (see, for example, Charmaz, 2000, 2006; Kelle, 2005; Locke, 1996; May, 1996; Mills, Bonner, & Francis, 2006). Like any other significant statement, followers may reify the version of grounded theory to which they subscribe and rigidify its tenets. Margaret H. Kearney (2007) has observed firsthand that Strauss's doctoral students clamored for more prescriptive rules than he wished to create.

Differences among current grounded theory proponents arise in the following areas: (1) epistemological allegiances, (2) methodological strategies that constitute grounded theory, (3) assumptions about what "theory," means, and (4) conceptual directions.[8] I have dealt extensively with methodological strategies (Charmaz, 2003, 2006, 2007c) and assumptions about theory (Charmaz, 2006) elsewhere but will take up differences in epistemological allegiances and suggest differences in conceptual directions here. Thus, this chapter continues and advances the epistemological explication and critique of grounded theory that I initiated in 1990 and have developed since then (Bryant & Charmaz, 2007a; Charmaz, 2000, 2002a, 2005, 2006, 2007a, 2007b, 2008a, 2008b, 2008c).

Most epistemological differences remain unstated in our empirical analyses but may become manifest in the kinds of data we collect and how we render them. Do the differences matter? Yes, they do. They matter in framing the range of our empirical observations, the theoretical depth and reach of our analyses, and how we position them.

In short, shifting the grounds of grounded theory to a constructivist approach fosters renewal and revitalization of the method by integrating recent methodological developments with the original classic statement of the method. The constructivist approach challenges the assumption of creating general abstract theories and leads us to situated knowledges (Haraway, 1991), while simultaneously moving grounded theory further into interpretive social science.

The Movement of the Method: Grounded Theory in Process

Grounded theory is a method to study process. It is, moreover, a method *in* process. I underscore this point because we don't need to think of grounded theory as fixed and static. Indeed, it hasn't been fixed and static. Like qualitative inquiry more generally, grounded theory has shifted over the years. Anselm Strauss and Juliet Corbin (1990, 1998) are not the only ones who altered grounded theory. I've shifted the assumptions separately and together with Antony Bryant, who also shifted them separately and with me (Bryant, 2002, 2003; Bryant & Charmaz, 2007a, 2007b; Charmaz, 2000, 2002b, 2006, 2007a). Adele Clarke (2005, 2006, 2007) has shared this shift—and has moved the analysis of empirical situations further into organizational and societal discourses and structures.

Which grounded theory practices form the core of the method? To what extent is grounded theory a method of application or a method for innovation? What constitutes a grounded theory study? Everyone has reconstructed grounded theory, including Barney Glaser (Charmaz, 2008c). As I have pointed out before, Glaser has, however, maintained a remarkably consistent *logic* over the years. He has abandoned the search for a basic social process that distinguished the early grounded theory texts because he came to see it as forcing data into a preconceived framework (Glaser, 2001). He has also discarded the practice of line-by-line coding in favor of incident-by-incident coding because he believes line-by-line coding generates a jumble of unconnected codes. Glaser has talked of the continuing evolution of grounded theory, meaning classic grounded theory as he conceives it. Recently, however, he has become open to variations (Bryant & Charmaz, 2007b). Whether a particular variant of grounded theory has developed, shifted, eroded, or irrevocably changed grounded theory depends on what you define as the genuine method and on your epistemological perspective.

Consistent with grounded theory's comparative logic, the meaning of constructivist grounded theory becomes clearer if we compare its fundamental assumptions and logic with those of objectivist grounded theory.

To make these comparisons, we need to return to the original statement of the method and then ask: How does constructivist grounded theory compare with Glaser and Strauss's classic statement of grounded theory? Where do the continuities and discontinuities lie?

Objectivist and Constructivist Grounded Theory

As a heuristic device, it may be helpful to view objectivist and grounded theory as located on two ends of a continuum. My intent here is to clarify, not to reify a distinction. When we reify a phenomenon, in this case, a method, we take something that is a process and treat it as a rigid, concrete, and fixed structure. Using grounded theory is a process; the method itself is in process. Its fluidity and flexibility inhere in the method itself.

Both objectivist and constructivist grounded theory share certain assumptions and directions and differ on others. In practice, the lines between the two types may blur. Grounded theory in its constructivist version is a profoundly *interactive* method (Charmaz, 2000, 2006).[9] It emphasizes interaction throughout the analytic process as well as during data collection.

Constructivist grounded theory adopts the inductive, comparative, emergent, and open-ended approach of Glaser and Strauss's classic version. It also includes the abductive logic that Strauss emphasized in his early teaching but only noted in his 1987 text. Grounded theorists borrow the iterative logic of abduction to check and refine the development of categories. In brief, abductive reasoning follows inductive inquiry and takes it further. When a grounded theorist encounters a surprising finding while engaging in research, he or she (1) considers all conceivable theoretical ideas that could account for the finding, (2) returns to the field and gathers more data to put these ideas to test, and (3) subsequently, adopts the most plausible theoretical interpretation (Charmaz, 2006; Peirce, 1958; Reichert, 2007; Rosenthal, 2004). Abductive reasoning arises from experience, leads to logical but creative inferences, and invokes testing these inferences with hypotheses to arrive at a plausible theoretical explanation of experience.

The classic approach to abduction (Peirce, 1958; Reichert, 2007; Rosenthal 2004); starts with a surprising finding but grounded theorists also use an iterative approach when accounting for intriguing findings and checking their emergent categories. The concept of abduction clarifies that grounded theorists study their observations and develop abstractions about which they form working hypotheses to test against new observations (Atkinson, Delamont, & Coffey, 2003). Abduction offers a way of conceptualizing and working with data that fosters and guides the researcher's efforts to develop creative interpretations of studied life. Thus, abductive reasoning acknowledges both the pragmatist emphasis on a researcher's creative conceptualizations and the significance of his or her experience in formulating them (see Peirce, 1958).

Perhaps ironically, abduction comes closer to Glaser's emphasis on emergence in checking categories than Strauss and Corbin's application procedure of axial coding. Grounded theory begins with inductive analyses of data but moves beyond induction to create an imaginative interpretation of studied life. We adopt abductive logic when we engage in imaginative thinking about intriguing findings and then return to the field to check our conjectures. Hence, abduction underlies the iterative process of moving back and forth between data and conceptualization that characterizes grounded theory.

As we place objectivist and constructivist grounded theory on a continuum, we can compare their foundational assumptions, foci of analysis, and implications for conducting data analysis (see also Bryant, 2002; Charmaz, 2000, 2006) (see Figure 6.1). Objectivist grounded theory arises from positivism and thus assumes discovery of data in an external world by a neutral, but expert observer whose conceptualizations arise from the data. Data are separate facts from the observer and, in the objectivist view, should be observed without preconception.

In contrast, constructivist grounded theory reflects its pragmatist roots and relativist epistemology. Constructivist grounded theory assumes multiple realities—and multiple perspectives on these realities. Data are not separate from either the viewer or the viewed. Instead, they are mutually constructed through interaction. Granted, the grounded theorist renders these data but they arise in situations under particular conditions and therefore affect the resulting analysis. Thus, constructivist grounded theorists see the representation of data—and by extension, the analysis—as problematic, relativistic, situational, and partial.

The objectives of each approach flow from its foundational assumptions. Objectivists focus on developing abstract generalizations free from the contexts of their origins. Objectivists aim for parsimonious abstract explanations in a theory that fits the studied empirical data, works to explain them, has relevance to the research participants, and is modifiable.

Figure 6.1 Epistemological Underpinnings of Grounded Theory

Positivist	Pragmatist
Assumes *the* scientific method	Takes a problem-solving approach
Presupposes *an* external reality	Views reality as fluid, somewhat indeterminate
Assumes an unbiased observer	Assumes a situated and embodied knowledge producer
Assumes discovery of abstract generalities	Assumes search for multiple perspectives
Aims to explain empirical phenomena	Aims to study people's actions to solve emergent problems
Views facts and values as separable	Sees facts and values as co-constitutive
Views truth as conditional	Views truth as conditional

Constructivists, however, view generalizations as partial, conditional, and situated in time, space, positions, actions, and interactions. Constructivists aim for an interpretive understanding of the empirical phenomena in a theory that has credibility, originality, resonance, and usefulness, relative to its historical moment.

These foundational assumptions and objectives are played out in the respective foci of each approach. Objectivist grounded theory focuses on developing abstractions and invokes a variable analysis with a concept-indicator logic to explicate a core category or basic social process in the data (see Glaser, 1978, 1998). Hence, the researcher develops the category inductively from instances in the data, treats this category as a concept, and specifies its indicators. Objectivist grounded theory emphasizes overt statements and behavior. The objectivist looks at the empirical world from the outside as a visitor who does not enter the world of the research participants.[10]

Constructivists enter the empirical world to the extent that they can. They interpret the data through an emergent conceptual analysis of them. They seek to find the range of variation in their data and analyses and look for relationships between their emerging categories. As constructivists engage their data, they focus on liminal meanings and tacit actions as well as explicit statements and actions.

Not surprisingly, the different foci have implications for the practice of doing data analysis. Objectivists treat data analysis as an objective process that they achieve by making their generalizations successively more abstract through comparative analysis. In Glaser's (2002) view, whatever bias the grounded theorist might have brought to the data is neutralized through making comparisons and by raising the level of abstraction of the categories. This logic assumes that comparing data with data, data with categories, and categories with categories build significant checks on a grounded theorist's biases. I agree, particularly if the grounded theorist is reflexive about the comparative process as well as the emerging categories. In the objectivist view, however, reflexivity could simply add another variable or source of data for abstraction rather than constitute an integral part of the entire research process. From an objectivist perspective, the grounded theorist's training and comparative analytic rigor grants him or her legitimacy and authority to make claims of objectivity.

Constructivists not only acknowledge the relativity of the data but also that subjectivities enter the analysis as well as data collection. Rather than denying their existence and donning the cloak of the objective scientist, constructivists argue for explicating how their standpoints, positions, situations, and interactions have influenced their analytic renderings. Such explication is not easy and may arise in part from colleagues or research participants' tough questions, as Casper (1997) experienced. From a constructivist view, the analysis is conditional, contingent, and partial. Abstract understanding does not render generalization objective. Instead, it erases the contingencies and relativity inherent in inquiry and the differences and variation in social life, as Adele Clarke has extensively detailed (2005, 2006, 2007).

When we look at the foundational assumptions in objectivist and constructivist grounded theory, the fit between pragmatism and constructivist grounded theory is striking (see Figure 6.2). Pragmatism assumes a multiplicity of perspectives, views reality as consisting of emergent processes, addresses how people handle practical problems in their worlds, and sees facts and values as joined. All these dimensions reveal the congruence between pragmatism and constructivist grounded theory.

In which directions does a constructivist approach take us? The constructivist turn in grounded theory takes what is "real" as problematic

Figure 6.2
Objectivist Grounded Theory ➔ — ◆ *Constructivist Grounded Theory*

Comparisons and Contrast

Foundational Assumptions	Foundational Assumptions
Assumes an external reality.	Assumes multiple realities.
Assumes discovery of data.	Assumes mutual construction of data through interaction.
Assumes conceptualizations emerge from data.	Assumes researcher constructs categories.
Views representation of data as unproblematic.	Views representation of data as problematic, relativistic, situational, and partial.
Assumes the neutrality, passivity, and authority of the observer.	Assumes the observer's values, priorities, positions, and actions affect views.
Objectives	**Objectives**
Aims to achieve context-free generalizations.	Views generalizations as partial, conditional, and situated in time, space, positions, action, and interactions.
Aims for parsimonious, abstract conceptualizations that transcend historical and situational locations.	Aims for interpretive understanding of historically situated data.
Specifies variables.	Specifies range of variation.
Aims to create theory that fits, works, has relevance, and is modifiable. (Glaser)	Aims to create theory that has credibility, originality, resonance, and usefulness.
Implications for Data Analysis	**Implications for Data Analysis**
Views data analysis as an objective process.	Acknowledges subjectivities throughout data analysis.
Sees emergent categories as forming the analysis.	Recognizes co-construction of data shapes analysis.
Sees reflexivity as one possible data source.	Engages in reflexivity.
Gives priority to researcher's analytic categories and voice.	Seeks and (re)represents participants' views and voices as integral to the analysis.

in a way that I believe many grounded theorists do not. By taking what is real as problematic, constructivists go two steps back from classic grounded theory and simultaneously take a large step forward into interpretive social science. We go back to look at the multiple definitions of a given reality and how people enact that reality—in tacit as well as overt ways. We also see our views of their views and actions as problematic—a construction. By doing so, we question how our sensibilities and standpoints shape the realities that we see and define.

In keeping with its pragmatist heritage, constructivists pay close attention to language and look for the taken-for-granted properties of key terms and the assumptions on which these terms rest. For example, if we conducted a study on achievement in an elementary school, we would study what achievement meant to various participants, how they viewed it, and what their actions in regard to it assumed. We would try to break open our participants' presuppositions about achievement and scrutinize our own—and define it according to what we see as its fundamental properties. More commonly, grounded theorists start with the topic at hand as a given, not as an area to probe.

Constructivists attend to how people draw on socially constructed discourses. A discourse may be subtle and unstated because it is assumed. That's why the constructivist approach leads us to look at liminal, tacit meanings. In the example above, American discourse on educational achievement focuses on the individual, assumes the legitimacy of certain measures, not others, and takes into account a narrow range of areas.

The situated nature of past and immediate experience becomes grist for constructivists' analytic mill. Constructivists examine how experience is constituted.[11] Classic grounded theorists talk *about* experience from the outside more than getting inside the experience and taking it apart (Charmaz, 2006). By claiming a value-free stance, objectivists eliminate the problematic messiness inherent in inquiry rather than eradicating their preconceptions.[12] This messiness can become pressing when researchers hold explicit standpoints toward their topics and realize that their standpoints are consequential. Monica Casper (1997) demonstrates this messiness in her methodological reflection. She writes:

> As I continued to deal with the implications of taking sides in research, I found myself secretly longing for some Enlightenment objectivity, an epistemological shortcut out of these conundrums. Striving to be methodologically accountable to informants is hard

enough work; layering political accountability on top of that only deepens the contradictions. In a research site inhabited by a disparate group of informants with different perspectives, it is not surprising that my accountability took shape in various ways. Another researcher in this field might well have developed entirely different networks of accountability. Although I followed all the basic methodological rules of qualitative research, in terms of political accountability there seemed to be no basic rules. Figuring out how to manage my commitments on the reproductive frontier required tremendous effort. In the process, I discovered that choosing to be a research cowgirl is not without its costs. Yet I firmly believe that taking sides is worth this effort if our only alternative is to retreat into the hollow position of "objective" analyst. There are no epistemological shortcuts without a price. As Donna Haraway has written, "feminists have to insist on a better account of the world." (1997, pp. 251–252)

Constructivist grounded theory encourages the researcher to examine the standpoints of the participants, their historical locations, and social circumstances. How might we do that? I offer a short example from an analysis of grief titled, "Grief and Loss of Self" (Charmaz, 1997). Experiencing grief may seem like the most personal and subjective of experiences. It is. Yet it also means something more and different than solely subjective experience. Grief occurs within social life, and people draw on a shared language, rules, and traditions, not only for expressing it but, moreover, for experiencing it.[13] Grief reflects attachments and their meaning. In the following excerpt, I examine the discourse of what I call "entitled grief."

> Narrow American definitions of significant and worthy relationships grant certain bereaved *entitled grief* and priority status. Entitled grief is legitimate, deserved, expected, and, typically, obligatory sorrow over loss. Entitled grief affords its possessor a priority status—this survivor is seen as the deceased's closest kin. Righteous entitlement to express grief (within limits) accompanies the bereaved's justified priority in the hierarchy of loss. Deaths of spouses, especially young and middle-aged spouses, and children grant greatest entitlement and highest priority status. (Charmaz, 1997, p. 235)

How does the analysis above reflect constructivist grounded theory? Note that I defined the category "entitled grief" by its taken-for-granted properties. I pieced together what people said and did and looked for their implied meanings. In this way, a constructivist goes beneath the surface and enters the liminal world of meaning. My overall analysis of grief took me into the meanings of loss, into the dominant way North Americans define grief, and into the nature of the social bond and forms of attachment. What does grief tell us about social bonds, about attachment? North Americans view those who share close relationships with the bereaved as suffering loss and entitled to grieve—for a while. Here, people grant objective meaning to subjective experience. Thus, the most bereaved can make claims of entitlement at the time of the death and for a period afterward.

When we seek to learn *how* people construct meanings, we can discover *which* meanings they hold and how these meanings might answer the question of *what* our emerging category is about. The category, entitled grief, is both hierarchical and comparative. It places the legitimacy of grief in hierarchical order and assumes social roles, rights, and obligations. North Americans presuppose that the structural order of earlier role relationships with the deceased hierarchically order both survivors claims to deep grief and searing loss and shape their obligations to grieve. This view may remain unstated and unquestioned yet shape individuals' attitudes and actions.

My conceptual category, entitled grief, clearly compares the legitimacy and obligations of the next-of-kin with those whose place in the structure of relationships appears more removed. Although I use this category here for purposes of illustration, constructivists aim to identify the range and positioning of our categories. You might ask how entitled grief fits with other categories.[14] The category of entitled grief also compares with other types of grief, most explicitly, Kenneth Doka's (1989) insightful concept of "disenfranchised grief." Doka realized that North Americans do not define all grief as legitimate and that deep grief may go unacknowledged or unrecognized and thus remain invisible. Disenfranchised grief arises when a bereaved survivor receives no honor or privilege or rights relative to his or her loss, despite having or having had an intimate relationship with the deceased. Significant actors who control what happens after the death overlook this survivor should they know about him or her at all. Troubled or complicated relationships with and/or beyond the deceased set the conditions for certain individuals to later experience disenfranchised grief. Thus, this type of grief arises after a traumatic parting such as a hostile divorce, during a secret relationship such as an extra-marital affair, or when relatives make intentional or unintentional decisions that exclude a significant survivor such as those made by parents who have denied or rejected their adult child's homosexuality.

Both terms, "disenfranchised grief" and "entitled grief," are framed in telling metaphors that speak to wider cultural values that permeate people's consciousness and actions, often without their awareness. I had developed the idea of entitled grief over ten years before publication of my paper on grief (Charmaz, 1997) and later discovered that newly widowed screenwriter Stephanie Ericsson's (1993) reflection illustrated it. Ericsson had an acquaintance who mentioned understanding what she was experiencing because of having lost a parent two years before. Ericsson states thinking:

> [S]chmuck, that's supposed to happen, it's a natural part of becoming adult—children are supposed to outlive their parents. Did you lose the only other person in the world who would love your child the way you do? Did you lose the person you held all night, who slept next to you, warmed your bed so much you didn't need an extra blanket in the winter? ... Don't reduce this experience to something logical, universal. Even if it is, I walk alone amongst the dead, it's my death, my pain. Don't pretend you know it like you know my batting averages. Don't sacrilege all over my crucifixion. (p. 212)

Observe that while making claims of entitlement, Ericsson effectively lays out grounds for disenfranchising the grief of other people. In my published analysis of the type of grief that Ericsson's statement reflects, I wrote:

> Assumptions of entitled grief and priority status give rise to moral claims, as Ericsson reveals. Her grief permits claims of injustice, prompts claims of broken conventions of sensitivity, reaffirms the hierarchical ordering of loss, and, thus, fosters disattending to the losses of others. Sympathy may righteously be withheld. Here, the meaning of loss is predicated on objective structural relationships, not subjectively experienced ones. Entitled grief allows dramatizing one's own loss and minimizing the meaning of other people's "lesser" relationships. Entitled grief then gives license to focus on self. One turns inward perhaps even as one lashes outward. (Charmaz, 1997, p. 236)

Conclusion

A constructivist grounded theory can take us deep into the phenomena without isolating it from its social locations. Going deep into the phenomenon allows us to gain intimate knowledge of it and to work inductively from this position. It means going beyond scanty data collection and superficial analyses. Intimate knowledge provides us with a different location to understand studied life than those who remain outside it can attain. Going deep into the studied phenomenon prompts us to go to the roots of the issues we study. For example, I tried to define essential properties of entitled grief, as given in individuals' take-for-granted assumptions. Monica Casper (1998) tried to delineate the assumptions the fetal surgeons held about their clients and about their practice.

We can use grounded theory strategies to help us define essential properties and relationships when we go deep into studied life and yet connect it with larger concerns, as Casper's study exemplifies. She entered the world of the fetal surgeons and scrutinized their construction of meanings and actions but she never lost sight of larger questions about power, reproductive rights, and the quality of life. Through adopting the logic of this kind of inquiry, we can gain new views and challenge old assumptions while understanding the ambiguity inherent in inquiry and the messiness of the process.

In my view, the objectivist admonition to tolerate ambiguity lends tacit acknowledgment to the elusiveness of social phenomena and the interpretive nature of qualitative analysis. The "it" we take apart is seldom something so concrete and tangible that everyone views it from the same starting point and standpoint. Accepting the notions of a multiplicity of perspectives and multiple realities forces us to construct layered analyses and to attend to varied ways both we and our participants construct meaning.

Thus, relevant social locations arise during the course of inquiry as well as those clearly identifiable before entering the field setting. In this sense, constructivist grounded theory offers possibilities of simultaneously situating our studies, increasing the acuity of our analyses, and broadening their implications. By shifting the ontological and epistemological grounds of grounded theory now, we can construct the foundation for the next generation of grounded theorists to advance qualitative inquiry.

Acknowledgments

Many thanks are due to Janice Morse for her innovative idea of bringing second-generation grounded theorists together and making both the grounded theory conference and this volume possible. I thank Corrine D'Souza and Dori Fortune for their help in bringing both projects to fruition. No writing project is entirely solitary. I appreciate having had conversations about grounded theory over the years with Antony Bryant, César Cisneros-Puebla, Adele Clarke, Ray Maietta, Janice Morse, and Virginia Olesen and am indebted to Dorothy Freidel, Diana Grant, Matthew James, Josh Meisel, Melinda Milligan, and Richard Senghas, members of the Sonoma State University Faculty Writing Program, for commenting on an earlier version of this chapter. Special thanks are due to Adele Clarke for her excellent substantive comments and editorial suggestions on a later version of this chapter.

Notes

1. I consider Glaser *and* Strauss's first exegesis of grounded theory in the *Discovery* book and Glaser's (1978) subsequent statement in *Theoretical Sensitivity* to represent the classic statements of the method.

2. Kath Melia (see 1987, 1996) stands as notable exception. Unlike most early doctoral students who became proponents of grounded theory, she studied with neither Glaser nor Strauss. She adopted Glaser's (1978) *Theoretical Sensitivity* as a guide for conducting her research and produced a dissertation and excellent book (1987) remarkably congruent with grounded theory logic.

3. Studies of science and technology have long found that scientific methods vary and are contingent on local practices. Thus unitary methods do not exist in concrete practices only in claims-making about methods (personal communication, Adele Clarke, January 15, 2008).

4. Interestingly, Glaser (1991) acknowledges learning lessons from Strauss that later became hallmarks of Glaserian grounded theory such as (1) build theory from data; (2) look for what is happening in the field setting; (3) see one's empirically grounded ideas as what counts, not the data; and (4) guard against forcing the data into preconceived categories.

5. I am not faulting researchers who do not discuss how they have affected the research process. Scholarly journals focus on original research, not research accounts. Journal traditions emphasize data collection techniques and samples rather than reflections in the methods sections of their respective articles. Book publishers may limit—or eliminate—pages for methodological discussions. Relatively few qualitative researchers and even fewer grounded theorists among them have written detailed discussions about how their studies evolved. In the past, venues for such discussions have been rather limited, but now more journals and edited volumes publish methodological essays that bring reflexivity into public discourse.

6. "Studying up" (Nader 1972) not only poses access problems in locating settings and individuals but also poses access problems within settings and with powerful elite individuals who control these settings. Elites exist within networks and can help or hinder researchers to gain access to the network. Elites also can set the conditions of interaction with the researcher by controlling contact and conversation with him or her. As Casper (1998) discovered, losing access from elites can also mean losing access to all other potential participants for whom these elites serve as gatekeepers. For ideas about studying up, see Kezar (2003), Nader (1997), Odendahl and Shaw (2002), Ostrander (1993), and Stephens (2007).

7. Another unrecognized problem arises with critics who do not use the method but issue pronouncements about it. The generality of their criticisms not only appears to encompass all variants of grounded theory but typically also

lacks specific evidence on which readers can assess their claims. Authoritative figures whose authoritative knowledge does not extend to grounded theory can mislead seasoned researchers as well as novices.

8. See also (Bryant & Charmaz, 2007a, 2007b; Charmaz, 2006; Clarke, 2005, 2006; Clarke & Friese, 2007; Kelle, 2005; May, 1996; Mills, Bonner, & Francis, 2006; Walker & Myrick, 2006) for further discussion of these differences.

9. In his critique of my position, Glaser (2002) correctly identified the significance of interaction in constructivist grounded theory but viewed it as part of an agenda to produce accurate data. In response to my contention that we interpret data in our very selection and recording of it, Glaser argues that interaction and interpretation signify the unnecessary intrusion of the researcher.

10. Because of the researcher's status as a visitor and distanced relationship with research participants, objectivist grounded theory raises anew the implications of an underlying colonialist and imperialist mentality that anthropologists have confronted. I am indebted to Adele Clarke for emphasizing this point (personal communication, January 5, 2008). See also Clifford and Marcus (1986) and Marcus and Fischer (1986).

11. I am using the term "experience" broadly here. Clarke (2005) argues that social life consists of situations. We can not only look at those situations that arise in immediate interaction but also address those that are enacted as part of relatively stable structures. Both Clarke and I aim to take into account silences (Charmaz, 2002, 2008d; Clarke, 2003, 2005, 2006).

12. In his classic positivist statement, Emile Durkheim (1895/1982) made the dictum, "eradicate preconceptions" the first rule of the sociological method. Since then, the notion of value-free inquiry has rested on researchers eradicating their preconceptions.

13. See Arlie Hochchild's (1979) statement on feeling rules.

14. The utility of grounded theory works can also bring our category into policy discussions. Although the fetal surgeons Casper (1998) studied took umbrage about her work, fetal surgeons at another major medical center read her book, engaged her ideas, and invited her to participate in a conference with them (personal communication, February 11, 2008).

References

Atkinson, P., Coffey, A., & Delamont, S. (2003). *Key themes in qualitative research: Continuities and changes.* New York: Roman & Littlefield.

Bowker, G. & Star, S. L. (1999). *Sorting things out: Classification and its consequences.* Cambridge, MA: MIT Press.

Boychuk Duchscher, J. E. & Morgan, D. (2004). Grounded theory: Reflections on the emerging vs. forcing debate. *Journal of Advanced Nursing,* 48(6), 605–612.

Bryant, A. (2002). Re-grounding grounded theory. *Journal of Information Technology Theory and Application,* 4(1), 25–42.

Bryant, A. (2003). A constructive/ist response to Glaser. *FQS: Forum for Qualitative Social Research,* 4(1). Available online at www.qualitative-research.net/fqs/-texte/1-03/1-03bryant-e.htm (accessed March 14, 2003).

Bryant, A. & Charmaz, K. (2007a). Grounded theory in historical perspective: An epistemological account. In A. Bryant & K. Charmaz (Eds.), *The handbook of grounded theory* (pp. 31–57). London: Sage.

Bryant, A. & Charmaz, K. (2007b). Introduction. In A. Bryant & K. Charmaz (Eds.), *Handbook of grounded theory* (pp. 1–28). London: Sage.

Burawoy, M. (1991). The extended case method. In M. Burawoy, J. Gamson, J. Schiffman, A. Burton, A. A. Ferguson, L. Salzinger, S. Ui, L. Hurst, & K. Fox (Eds.), *Ethnography unbound: Power and resistance in the modern metropolis* (pp. 271–290). Berkeley: University of California Press.

Casper, M. J. (1997). Feminist politics and fetal surgery: Adventures of a research cowgirl on the reproductive frontier. *Feminist Studies,* 23(2), 232–262.

Casper, M. J. (1998). *The making of the unborn patient: A social anatomy of fetal surgery.* New Brunswick, NJ: Rutgers University Press.

Charmaz, K. (1990). Discovering chronic illness: Using grounded theory. *Social Science & Medicine,* 30, 1161–1172.

Charmaz. K. (1997). Grief and loss of self. In K. Charmaz, G. Howarth, & A. Kellehear (Eds.), *The unknown country: Death in Australia, Britain and the U.S.A.* (pp. 229–241). London: Macmillan.

Charmaz. K. (2000). Constructivist and objectivist grounded theory. In N. K. Denzin & Y. S. Lincoln (Eds.), *Handbook of qualitative research,* 2nd ed. (pp. 509–535). Thousand Oaks, CA: Sage.

Charmaz, K. (2002a). Grounded theory analysis. In J. F. Gubrium and J. A. Holstein (Eds.), *Handbook of interview research* (pp. 675–694). Thousand Oaks, CA: Sage.

Charmaz. K. (2002b). Stories and silences: Disclosures and self in chronic illness. *Qualitative Inquiry,* 8, 302–328.

Charmaz, K. (2003). Grounded theory. In J. A. Smith (Ed.), *Qualitative psychology: A practical guide to research methods* (pp. 81–110). London: Sage.

Charmaz, K. (2005). Grounded theory in the 21st century: A qualitative method for advancing social justice research. In N. Y. Denzin & Y. S. Lincoln (Eds.), *Handbook of qualitative research*, 3rd ed. (pp. 507–535). Thousand Oaks, CA: Sage.

Charmaz, K. (2006). *Constructing grounded theory: A practical guide through qualitative analysis.* London: Sage.

Charmaz, K. (2007a). Constructionism and the grounded theory method. In J. A. Holstein and J. F. Gubrium (Eds.), *Handbook of constructionist research* (pp. 397–412). New York: Guilford.

Charmaz, K. (2007b). Grounded theory. In Jonathan A. Smith (Ed.), *Qualitative psychology: A practical guide to research methods* (pp. 82–110). London: Sage.

Charmaz, K. (2008a). Grounded theory as an emergent method. In S. Hesse-Biber & P. Leavy (Eds.), *The handbook of emergent methods* (pp. 155–170). New York: Guilford.

Charmaz, K. (2008b). The legacy of Anselm Strauss for constructivist grounded theory. In N. K. Denzin (Ed.), *Studies in Symbolic Interaction* (pp. 125–139). Bingley, UK: Emerald Publishing Group, Ltd.

Charmaz, K. (2008c). Reconstructing grounded theory. In L. Bickman, P. Alasuutari, & J. Brannen (Eds.), *Handbook of social research* (pp. 461–478). London: Sage.

Charmaz. K. (2008d). Stories and silences: Disclosures and self in chronic illness. In D. Brashers & D. Goldstein (Eds.), *Health communication.* New York: Lawrence Erlbaum.

Charmaz, K. & Henwood, K. (2008). Grounded theory in psychology. In C. Willig & W. Stainton-Rogers (Eds.), *Handbook of qualitative research in psychology.* London: Sage.

Cisneros-Puebla, C. A. (2007). The deconstructive and reconstructive faces of social construction. Kenneth Gergen in conversation with César A. Cisneros-Puebla. With an introduction by Robert B. Faux [83 paragraphs]. *Forum Qualitative Sozialforschung/Forum: Qualitative Social Research*, 9(1), Art. 20. Available online at http://www.qualitative-research.net/fqs-texte/1-08/08-1-20-e.htm (accessed August 31, 2007).

Clarke, A. E. 1998. *Disciplining reproduction: Modernity, American life sciences and the "problem of sex."* Berkeley: University of California Press.

Clarke, A. E. (2003). Situational analyses: Grounded theory mapping after the postmodern turn. *Symbolic Interaction*, 26(4), 553–576.

Clarke, A. E. (2005). *Situational analysis: Grounded theory after the postmodern turn.* Thousand Oaks, CA: Sage.

Clarke, A. E. (2006). Feminisms, grounded theory, and situational analysis. In S. Hess-Biber & D. Leckenby (Eds.), *Handbook of feminist research methods* (pp. 345–370). Thousand Oaks, CA: Sage.

Clarke, A. E. (2007). Grounded theory: Conflicts, debates and situational analysis. In W. Outhwaite & S. P. Turner (Eds.), *Handbook of social science methodology* (pp. 838–885). Thousand Oaks, CA: Sage.

Clarke, A. E. & Friese, C. (2007). Grounded theorizing: Using situational analysis. In A. Bryant and K. Charmaz (Eds.), *The handbook of grounded theory* (pp. 363–397). London: Sage.

Clifford, J. and Marcus, G. (Eds.). (1986). *Writing culture: The poetics and politics of ethnography*. Berkeley, CA: University of California Press.

Doka, K. J. (1989). Disenfranchised grief. In K. J. Doka (Ed.), *Disenfranchised grief: Recognizing hidden sorrow* (pp. 3–12). Lexington, MA: Lexington Books.

Durkheim, E. 1895/1982. *The rules of the sociological method*. Chicago: University of Chicago Press.

Ericsson, S. (1993). The agony of grief. In G. E. Dickinson, M. R. Leming, & A. C. Mermann (Eds.), *Dying, death, and bereavement* (pp. 210–212). Guilford, CT: Dushkin.

Fujimura, J. 1992. Crafting science: Standardized packages, boundary objects and "translation." In A. Pickering (Ed.), *Science as practice and culture* (pp. 168–214). Chicago: University of Chicago Press.

Glaser, B. G. (1978). *Theoretical sensitivity*. Mill Valley, CA: Sociology Press.

Glaser, B. G. (1991). In honor of Anselm Strauss: Collaboration. In D. R. Maines (Ed.), *Social organization and social process: Essays in honor of Anselm Strauss* (pp. 11–16). New York: Aldine de Gruyter.

Glaser, B. G. (1992). *Basics of grounded theory analysis*. Mill Valley, CA: Sociology Press.

Glaser, B. G. (1998). *Doing grounded theory: Issues and discussions*. Mill Valley, CA: Sociology Press.

Glaser, B. G. (2001). *The grounded theory perspective: Conceptualization contrasted with description*. Mill Valley, CA: Sociology Press.

Glaser, B. G. (2002). Constructivist grounded theory? Forum qualitative Sozialforschung/ Forum: *Qualitative Social Research* [on-line journal], 3. Available online at http://www.qualitative-research.net/fqs-texte/3-02/3-02glaser-e-htm (accessed February 23, 2003).

Glaser, B. G. & Strauss, A.L. (1967). *The discovery of grounded theory*. Chicago: Aldine.

Haraway, D. (1991). Situated knowledges: The science question in feminism and the privilege of partial perspective. In *Simians, cyborgs, and women: The reinvention of nature* (pp. 183–202). New York: Routledge.

Henwood, K. & Pidgeon, N. (2003). Grounded theory in psychological research. In P. M. Camic, J. E. Rhodes, & L. Yardley (Eds.), *Qualitative research in psychology: Expanding perspectives in methodology and design* (pp. 131–155). Washington, DC: American Psychological Association.

Karp, D. (1996). *Speaking of sadness: Depression, disconnection, and the meanings of illness.* New York: Oxford University Press.

Kearney, M. H. (2007). From the sublime to the meticulous: The continuing evolution of grounded formal theory. In A. Bryant & K. Charmaz (Eds.), *The handbook of grounded theory* (pp. 127–150). London: Sage.

Kelle, U. (2005). Emergence vs. forcing: A crucial problem of "grounded theory" reconsidered [52 paragraphs]. *Forum Qualitative Sozialforsung / Forum Qualitative Sociology* [on-line journal] 6, 2, Art. 27. Available online at http/www.qualitative-research.net/fqs.texte-2-05/05-2-27-e.htm (accessed May 30, 2005).

Kezar, A. (2003). Elite interviews: Missing link to transforming power relations. *Qualitative Inquiry* 9(3): 1–21.

Layder, D. (1998). *Sociological practice: Linking theory and social research.* London: Sage.

Locke, K. (1996). Rewriting the discovery of grounded theory after 25 years? *Journal of Management Inquiry,* 5(1), 239–245.

Marcus, G. & Fischer, R. (1986). *Anthropology as cultural critique: An experimental moment in the human sciences.* Chicago: University of Chicago Press.

May, K. (1996). Diffusion, dilution or distillation? The case of grounded theory method. *Qualitative Health Research,* 6(3), 309–311.

Mead, G. H. (1934). *Mind, self and society.* Chicago: University of Chicago Press.

Melia, K. M. (1987). *Learning and working: The occupational socialization of nurses.* London: Tavistock.

Melia, K. M. (1996). Rediscovering Glaser. *Qualitative Health Research,* 6(3), 368–378.

Mills, J., Bonner, A., & Francis, K. (2006). The development of constructivist grounded theory. *International Journal of Qualitative Methods,* 5(1), 1–10.

Nader, L. (1972). Up the anthropologist: Perspectives gained from studying up. In D. Hymes (Ed.), *Reinventing anthropology* (pp. 284–311). New York: Pantheon Books.

Nader, L. (1997). Controlling processes: Tracing the dynamic components of power. *Current Anthropology,* 38(5), 711–737.

Odendahl, Teresa and Aileen M. Shaw. 2002. Interviewing elites. In J. Gubrium and J. A. Holstein (Eds.) *Handbook of interview research: Context and method* (pp. 299–316). Thousand Oaks, CA: Sage.

Ostrander, Susan A. (1993). Surely you're not in this just to be helpful: Access, rapport, and interviews in three studies of elites. *Journal of Contemporary Ethnography,* 22 (1), 1–27.

Peirce, C. S. (1958). *Collected papers.* Cambridge: Harvard University Press.

Reichert, J. (2007). Abduction: The logic of discovery in grounded theory. In A. Bryant & K. Charmaz (Eds.), *The handbook of grounded theory* (pp. 214–228). London: Sage.

Rosenthal, G. (2004). Biographical research. In C. Seale, G. Gobo, J. F. Gubrium, & D. Silverman (Eds.), *Qualitative research practice* (pp. 48–64). London: Sage.

Star, S. L. (1989). *Regions of the mind: Brain research and the quest for scientific certainty.* Stanford, CA: Stanford University Press.

Star, S. L. & Griesemer, J. (1989). Institutional ecology, "translations" and boundary objects: Amateurs and professionals in Berkeley's Museum of Vertebrate Zoology, 1907–1939. *Social Studies of Science*, 19 (3), 387–420.

Stephens, N. (2007). Collecting data from elites and ultra elites: Telephone and face-to-face interviews with macroeconomists. *Qualitative Research*, 7(2), 203–216.

Strauss, A. L. (1987). *Qualitative analysis for social scientists.* New York: Cambridge University Press.

Strauss, A. L. & Corbin, J. (1990). *Basics of qualitative research: Grounded theory procedures and techniques.* Newbury Park, CA: Sage.

Strauss, A. L. & Corbin, J. (1994). Grounded theory methodology: An overview. In N. K. Denzin & Y. S. Lincoln (Eds.), *Handbook of qualitative research* (pp. 273–285). Newbury Park, CA: Sage.

Strauss, A. L. & Corbin, J. (1998). *Basics of qualitative research: Grounded theory procedures and techniques,* 2nd ed. Thousand Oaks, CA: Sage.

Walker, D. & Myrick, F. (2006). Grounded theory: An exploration of process and procedure. *Qualitative Health Research*, 16(4), 547–559.

Example: The Body, Identity, and Self

Adapting to Impairment

Kathy Charmaz

Chronic illness assaults the body and threatens the integrity of self. Having a serious chronic illness shakes earlier taken-for-granted assumptions about possessing a smoothly functioning body. It also disturbs a person's previous assumptions about the relation between body and self and disrupts a sense of wholeness of body and self (cf. Bury 1982; Brody 1987; Charmaz 1991; 1994a; 1994b; Gadow 1982; Monks and Frankenberg n.d.; Murphy 1987). Thus, chronic illness with impairment intrudes upon a person's daily life and undermines self and identity. What happens when people have chronic illnesses that weaken, challenge, or negate valued images of their bodies? How do beliefs, images, and expectations of one's body affect present identity and future hopes and plans? What kinds of goals do people form for their future identities after they have experienced loss of bodily function or disability?

To explicate how the body, identity, and self intersect in illness, I outline *one* mode of living with impairment or loss of bodily function: adapting. By adapting, I mean altering life and self to accommodate to physical losses and to reunify body and self accordingly. Adapting implies that the individual acknowledges impairment and alters life and self in socially and personally acceptable ways. Bodily limits and social circumstances often force adapting to loss. Adapting shades into acceptance. Thus, ill people adapt when they try to accommodate and flow with the experience of illness.

Other ways of living with illness include ignoring it, minimizing it, struggling against it, reconciling self to it, and embracing it (see Charmaz

1991; Radley 1991). People ignore and minimize illness when they do not experience its effects on their lives or can control those effects. They also ignore and minimize when other goals take precedence, such as keeping a job or attending to an intimate's needs. Through ignoring and minimizing, ill people may preserve the sense of unity between body and self that they had before illness. Preserving that unity becomes much harder when they constantly struggle against illness—they fight it and the identifications that come with it. Many people reconcile themselves to illness for years. They tolerate it—within limits. Hence, they define going beyond those limits such as "needing a wheelchair" or "going into a nursing home" as more than they can handle emotionally (see Charmaz 1991). When reconciling self to illness, people acknowledge and attempt working around it, but they neither accept it as defining them nor do they accept others' pronouncements of whom they now should be. In contrast, embracing illness means seeking refuge in it.

People with chronic illnesses often experience all these ways of living with impairment at different times. All may be necessary and natural responses to their experience, depending on their situations. After long years of ignoring, minimizing, struggling against, and reconciling themselves to illness, they adapt as they regain a sense of wholeness, of unity of body and self in the face of loss.

Modes of living with impairment are embedded in social definitions of "appropriate" *attitudes*, *actions*, and *activity levels*. Such judgments take into account *dependency* and *deviance*. Hence, negative definitions result when others view ill people as failing to reveal "correct" feelings or to take the "right" stance, engaging in "too much" or "too little" activity than physically warranted, becoming more independent or dependent than expected, or sinking into depression, drugs, or drunkenness. Some people never adapt to impairment; others refuse to admit that they have suffered losses (see examples in Albrecht 1992; Herzlich 1973; Radley and Green 1985; 1987; Williams 1981a; 1981b). Still others adapt to their impaired bodies only long after suffering losses. Many people, however, must adapt time and again as they progressively experience failing health, whether they slowly decline or rapidly plummet during acute episodes, crises, or complications. In whatever way people live with impairment, they prefer to have certain future identities over others, although their preferences may be wholly unattainable. Some chronically ill adults hold fast to regaining their unimpaired selves. Others pursue contradictory identities. For example, a stroke patient may simultaneously want to be the passive patient today and the fully recovered worker tomorrow without realizing that the latter requires concerted effort right now.

Adapting to an impaired body means resolving the tension between body and self elicited by serious chronic illness. It also means defining integration and wholeness of being while experiencing loss and suffering. These meanings of adapting to an impaired body become implicit criteria for "successful" adaptation with the taken-for-granted proviso that the person also remains as independent and autonomous as possible. Hence, successful adaptation means living with illness without living solely for it. Adapting to physical loss ebbs and flows and repeats itself in similar forms as further episodes, complications, and additional illnesses occur.

Studying adaptation to loss through impairment illuminates tensions within continuing metaphors of opposition[1]: the self versus the body, struggle versus surrender, the idealized body versus the real, experienced body, social identifications versus self-definitions, objective reality versus subjective experience, struggling with versus struggling against illness, invisible disability versus obvious impairment, freedom of bodily movement versus physical constraint and dependence, and bodily control versus loss of function. Though quelled before, these tensions reemerge with each disruptive episode or with deteriorating social conditions.

Adapting to impairment consists of three major stages. First, it depends upon experiencing an altered body, that in turn leads to defining impairment or loss and to making reassessments. Whether chronically ill people objectify their bodies and struggle against illness or subjectively integrate their ill bodies with self shapes whether or not they create a sense of wholeness of body and self and of their lives. Bodily appearance affects social identifications and self-definitions and, therefore, how an individual experiences an altered body. Second, assessing one's altered body, appearance to self and others, and the context of life results in changing one's future identity accordingly. Ill people make identity trade-offs, in other words, opting for one identity over another, as they weigh their situations and losses and gains. Even when forced to accept a lesser identity than previously, they often redefine their decisions as positive and find value in their restricted lives. Third, surrendering to the sick body means the end of the quest for control over illness. At this point, people open themselves to experiencing their illness; they define unity of body and self through this experience.

Theoretical Framework

This article takes a symbolic interactionist perspective on identity (Blumer 1969; Cooley 1902; Lindesmith, Strauss, and Denzin 1988; Mead 1934; and Strauss 1959) and builds upon the emerging literature on the body (DiGiacomo 1992; Frank 1990; 1991a; 1991b; Frankenberg 1990; Freund 1982; 1988; 1990; Gadow 1982; Glassner 1988; 1989; Kotarba 1994; Olesen 1994; Olesen, Schatzman, Droes, Hatton, and Chico 1990; Sanders 1990; Scheper-Hughes and Lock 1987; Zola 1982; 1991). I draw upon the philosopher Sally Gadow's (1982) clarification of the relation between body and self and on my earlier work on the self in chronic illness (Charmaz 1991) and the effects of loss upon identity (Charmaz 1987).

In keeping with symbolic interactionism, personal identity means the way an individual defines, locates, and differentiates self from others (see Hewitt 1992). Following Peter Burke (1980), the concept of identity implicitly takes into account the ways people *wish* to define themselves. Wishes are founded on feelings as well as thoughts. If possible, ill people usually try to turn their wishes into intentions, purposes, and actions. Thus, they are motivated to realize future identities, and are sometimes forced to acknowledge present ones. However implicitly, they form identity goals. Here, I define identity goals as *preferred identities* that people assume, desire, hope, or plan for (Charmaz 1987). The concept of identity goals assumes that human beings create meanings and act purposefully as they interpret their experience and interact within the world. Some people's identity goals are implicit, unstated, and understood; other people have explicit preferred identities. Like other categories of people, some individuals with chronic illnesses assume that they will realize their preferred identities; others keep a watchful eye on their future selves and emerging identities as they experience the present (see also, Radley and Green 1987).

Gadow (1982) assumes that human existence essentially means

embodiment and that the self is inseparable from the body. I agree. Mind and consciousness depend upon being in a body. In turn, bodily feelings affect mind and consciousness. Yet, as Gadow points out, body and self, although inseparable, are not identical. The relation between body and self becomes particularly problematic for those chronically ill people who realize that they have suffered lasting bodily losses. The problematic nature of such realizations intensifies for ill people who had previously pursued and preserved an endless youth through controlling and constructing their bodies (Turner 1992). Thus, meanings of loss are embedded in assumptions and discourses about the body. Not only do individuals assume bodily control through rational practices, but they also assume their practices achieve and, quite literally, embody individualism (Shilling 1993).

As Victor Kestenbaum (1982) observes, illness threatens a person's sense of integrity of self and the body and of self and the world. People who have serious chronic illnesses find progressive losses repeatedly threaten their body and self-integrity. They risk becoming socially identified and self-defined exclusively by their impaired bodies (Bury 1988; Goffman 1963; Locker 1983; MacDonald 1988). Thus, chronically ill people who move beyond loss and transcend stigmatizing negative labels define themselves as much more than their bodies and as much more than an illness (Charmaz 1991).

Gadow argues that illness and aging result in loss of the original unity of body and self and provide the means of recovering it at a new level. She assumes that an original unity existed and implies that loss and recovery of unity is a single process. However, what unity means can only be defined subjectively. Some people may not have defined themselves as having experienced such unity before illness, or as only having partially experienced it. Further, with each new and often unsuspected bodily impairment, people with chronic illnesses *repeatedly* experience loss of whatever unity between body and self they had previously defined or accepted. Thus, at each point when they suffer and define loss, identity questions and identity changes can emerge or reoccur. Throughout this article, I deal with the loss of body-self unity and its recovery through acknowledging bodily experience and opening oneself to the quest for harmony between body and self.

In order to understand how loss and recovery of body-self unity occurs, we must understand ill people's meanings of their bodily experiences and the social contexts in which they occur (Fabrega and Manning 1972; Gerhardt 1979; Radley and Green 1987; Zola 1991). Such meanings arise in dialectical relation to their biographies (Bury 1982; 1988; 1991; Corbin and Strauss 1987; 1988; Dingwall 1976; Gerhardt 1989; Radley 1989; Radley and Green 1987; Williams 1984) and are mediated by their interpretations of ongoing experiences. Consistent with symbolic interactionist social psychology, present meanings of the ill body and self develop from, but are not determined by, past discourses of meaning and present social identifications (Blumer 1969; Goffman 1963; Mead 1934).

As chronic illness encroaches upon life, people learn that it erodes their taken-for-granted preferred identities as well as their health. Further, they may discover that visible illness and disability can leave them with a master status and overriding stigmatized identity. Because of their physical losses, they reassess who they are and who they can become. Subsequently, they form identity goals as they try to reconstruct normal lives to whatever extent possible (Charmaz 1987; 1991). Frequently, people with chronic illnesses initially plan and expect to resume their lives unaffected by illness, or even to exceed their prior identity goals. As they test their bodies and themselves, ill people need to make identity trade-offs at certain points, or even to lower their identity goals systematically until they match their lessened capacities. At other times, they may gradually raise their hopes and progressively increase their identity goals when they meet with success. Therefore, both raised or lowered identity goals form an implicit identity hierarchy that ill people create as they adapt to bodily loss and change (Charmaz 1987).

Methods and Data

Grounded theory methods provided the strategies for collecting and analyzing data (Charmaz 1983; 1990; 1995; Glaser 1978; Glaser and Strauss 1967; Strauss 1987; Strauss and Corbin 1990; 1993). Consistent with the emergent character of grounded theory methods, my analysis evolved as I collected and interpreted data. While completing a study of the experience of chronic illness, I found that issues about having a problematic body arose repeatedly. This study included 115 intensive interviews of fifty-five adults with serious, intrusive chronic illnesses (cf. Charmaz 1991; Lofland and Lofland 1994; Seidman 1991). Sixteen of these respondents were followed longitudinally from five years to over a decade. After analyzing the earlier interviews for content about the body in illness, twenty-five additional highly focused interviews were conducted (including twelve interviews with respondents from the longitudinal portion of the original study) of two to three hours in length. I also collected personal accounts of experiencing chronic illness and disability to examine them for statements about the body (see, for example, Beisser 1988; Fisher, Straus, Cheney, and Oleske 1987; Frank 1990; LeMaistre 1985; Mairs 1989; Murphy 1987; Pitzele 1985; Register 1987). The first set of interviews stimulated my initial ideas about the body and self; the focused interviews elicited detailed information about the body and self, and the personal accounts provided independent sources of data for checking my ideas.

The respondents' characteristics varied by gender, age, and socioeconomic and diagnostic statuses. Two-thirds of the first set of respondents were middle-aged women (all respondents were over age twenty-one and white); two-thirds of the men were middle-aged; three-quarters of all respondents were working or middle-class. Two-thirds of those under age sixty worked part-time, full-time, or intermittently; other respondents quit work, attended school, went on disability, or retired early. Slightly over one-half of the respondents were married. Their chronic illnesses include heart and circulatory disease, cancer, emphysema, diabetes, chronic fatigue syndrome, rheumatoid and collagen diseases (arthritis, lupus erythematosus, Sjogren's syndrome, mixed connective tissue disease), and other auto-immune diseases such as multiple sclerosis. Almost one-third of the second sample of focused interviews were conducted with men. Except for one respondent in his twenties, respondents' ages ranged from forty to sixty (twelve respondents) and older, 61–75 years old. Half of all respondents were married; three were single; the remainder were divorced or separated. All were white.

I provide a stage analysis of adapting to impairment as a heuristic device to understand experiencing illness, not as an ultimate truth or as a prescriptive tool for practitioners and patients, as Elisabeth Kubler-Ross's

(1969) stage analysis proved to be. Depending on their physical condition and social resources, individuals may tumble through the stages rapidly and repeatedly, or they may plateau for years before moving into the next phase of adapting. A constructivist grounded theory perspective that emphasizes respondents' lived experience and stories (cf. Dawson and Prus 1992; Denzin 1988; Prus 1995) informs my analysis, rather than a more positivistic approach such as that of Anselm Strauss and Juliet Corbin (1990). The analytic steps included: (1) examining the first set of interviews and personal accounts for statements about the body, self, and identity, (2) developing themes around these topics that were explored in detail in the second set of interviews, (3) building analytic categories from the themes, and (4) linking the categories into a coherent process.

Experiencing an Altered Body

Experiencing an altered body means that people with illnesses note physical changes and diminished bodily functions (cf. Charmaz 1991; Kahane 1990; Kelly 1992; Yoshida 1993). Thus, experiencing an altered body means more than having or acquiring one. It means that these people begin to *define* bodily changes or the illness itself as real (if already diagnosed) and to account for how changes and symptoms affect daily life.[2] Distressing bodily sensations and impaired functions as well as disquieting feelings about body and self give rise to defining bodily changes. The unity of prior embodied experience has been shaken; assumptions about body and self have been jolted (see also, Olesen et al. 1990). At this point, people with illnesses compare their present body with their past body; they assess the differences between then and now, and they measure the costs and risks of ordinary activities. Before becoming ill, most people took their bodies for granted as functioning instruments or vehicles subjugated to the self. This taken-for-granted instrument becomes the yardstick against which they compare their altered bodies. A forty-one-year-old woman who had asthma described the bodily changes she experienced within the last year:

> By that time I really couldn't go for a walk, um, the way I used to, so I felt like my body had betrayed me. By that time I had, even though I hadn't really been diagnosed, I felt that even a little strain—I was

pushing myself and I knew it, you know. I knew that things that I used to do easily without any strain at all were a challenge. And so I was real aware of it. And also, probably at that time, I'd probably been running a low-grade fever for a long-time, and I knew it. . . . So I mostly felt like my body was sort of foreign territory—it was not the body that I knew.

Like others, this woman experienced her body as more than altered—she felt it was alien. Thus, she experienced a radical disruption of body and self. Experiencing this bodily alienation leads people to rethinking explicitly their previously held notions of body and self. This woman and several men with respiratory disease found that rapid weight gain accompanied plummeting physical activity. Mirror images of the body further call into question a previously taken-for-granted self. She said, "So I'm heavy—I'm heavy in a way I've never been before." Experiencing multiple bodily losses in a short period intensifies feelings of estrangement, of separation from one's past familiar body, and of loss of self. The body once viewed as a taken for granted possession to control and master has spun out of control. At best, the body is now a failed machine, an obstacle to be repaired, overcome, or mastered. At worst, it has become a deadly enemy or oppressor (cf. Charmaz 1980; 1994b; Gadow 1982; Herzlich 1973; Herzlich and Pierret 1984; Williams 1981a; 1981b).

When wholly unanticipated, even middle-aged people may view their bodily changes with a sense of betrayal. They may describe their past bodies as "invincible," "indestructible," and "immortal" and express regret and anger about their losses. In turn, their anger and regret intensify when ill people feel that their illnesses control them. They have lost control of their body as an object they assumed they could master. Moreover, they view themselves as overtaken by an alien force. The woman mentioned above stated:

It has probably slowed me down, and I'm very aware that I have this and if I really want to be as healthy as I can be, it's—it will control where I live; it will control what kind of work I do; it will control who I can be around—I can't be around someone who insists on wearing perfume; I can't be around anyone who smokes anything at all;

I can't be around people who insist on having … certain kinds of chemicals.

Perhaps more destructive than the anger is the guilt and shame followed by self-abasement that ill people with failing bodies experience: guilt because they share cultural standards of ageless bodily perfection and correct appearance (cf. Glassner 1988); shame because their very existence testifies to a failure to meet these standards. Self-abasement follows and intensifies the humiliation. Robert F. Murphy (1987, p. 111) observes:

> In my middle age, I had become a changeling, the lot of all disabled people. They are afflicted with a malady of the body that is translated into a cancer within the self and a disease of social relationships. They have experienced a transformation of the essential condition of their being in the world. They have become aliens, even exiles in their own lands.

For a time, people with chronic illnesses may make firm separations between their impaired bodies and their self-concepts (cf. Charmaz 1991; Register 1987; Weitz 1991). That way they can keep their illness separate from themselves and their lives. The extent to which they keep it separate and their stance about doing so is crucial. By keeping illness separate, they allay disquieting feelings about themselves and their bodies.

Struggling against illness differs from struggling with it. When people struggle *against* illness, they view their illness as the enemy with whom they must battle (cf. Charmaz 1980; 1994b). They hope to regain their past identities and to restore a now missing sense of self. Usually at this point, they can neither face nor accept more restricted lives and lesser identities than what they had before illness.

When people struggle *with* illness, they struggle to keep their bodies functioning and therefore, their lives "normal" to whatever extent possible. Hence, they do not give up. In struggling against and with illness, they try to take control over their illnesses and their bodies. Gregg Charles Fisher (1987, p. 13) describes how he and his wife struggled with chronic fatigue syndrome, implying that they learned to differentiate between body and self, despite their struggles: "Through the long years of this illness, we have had to struggle every day to cope with our affliction.

As the years go by, we are more determined than ever to remain strong. The saying that time heals all wounds is true, not because wounds, like sand castles, wash away with the first tide but because in time you learn to survive your wounds."

Through struggling with illness, these people eventually integrate new bodily facts into their lives and their self-concepts (cf. Charmaz 1991; Corbin and Strauss 1987). But until they define the changes as chronic and experience their effects daily, ill people look for recovery and can keep illness and therefore their bodies at the margins of their self-concepts (Charmaz 1991; 1994a). Subsequently, they continue to objectify their bodies and distance themselves from them.[3] Not only do their bodies become objects to mend but they are also worksites in which to do it. The situation differs for people who have already struggled with bodily oddities or "psychological" quirks now redefined and legitimated as bona fide physical symptoms. Their initial diagnostic relief turns into the sobering experience of adopting their medical label and of defining what it means to them. As they do so, they may make the label their own while simultaneously objectifying their symptoms that fit the diagnostic label. The writer Nancy Mairs (1989, pp. 235–236) redefines herself and her body as a woman with multiple sclerosis but also objectifies her body:

> Now I am who I will be. A body in trouble. I've spent all these years trying alternately to repudiate and to control my wayward body, to transcend it one way or another, but MS [multiple sclerosis] rams me right back down into it. "The body," I've gotten into the habit of calling it. "The left leg is weak," I say. "There's a blurred spot in the right eye." As though it were some other entity, remote and traitorous. Or worse, as though it were inanimate, a prison of bone, the dark tower around which Childe Roland rode, withershins left, withershins right, seeking to free the fair kidnapped princess: me.

The horror of the unknown—disability and death—prompts the distancing inherent in objectification. Distancing continues as long as the person assumes that mastering his or her wayward body is necessary to make it acceptable. Relinquishing notions of mastering one's body, in contrast, allows a receptivity to bodily experience. Arthur Frank (1991, pp. 60–61) reveals the moment when he shifted from objectifying his body to embracing it as subject: "I wondered at what the body could still do for me, as diseased as I knew it must be. That day I stopped resenting 'it' for the pain I had felt and began to appreciate my body, in some ways for the first time in my life. I stopped evaluating my body and began to draw strength from it. And I recognized that this body was me."

As ill people objectify their bodies less, they are more open to attending to the cues their bodies provide. They learn how to protect their bodies and therefore are able to extend their control over their lives. For example, a woman with lupus erythematosus learned that she could work at home while she was sick. At home, she could control the temperature, light, seating, and interruptions, as well as the pacing of her tasks. When she worked at her clients' offices, she could control little of that. She said:

> But see, I've always gone to the client's place to do the work and now, when I don't feel good, I'm finding that it's much easier to do it here at the house. And then I can just do—I can just do it at night; I can do it early in the morning. Yeah it's too hard to go and sit—sometimes the chairs they make me sit on or the—and it's too cold or it's too hot, or it's just real hard. I don't have the patience I used to have. I lost that. I used to have a lot of patience; I could bear anything. I don't think I was even aware of it. But now my body tells me. I can't control my body.

Before her illness, this woman had ignored bodily discomfort. At that time, she had committed herself, not only to a demanding work and social life but also to a rigorous fitness routine. She had pushed her body to be slim, strong, and taut, as she put it, "like a jungle tiger." She had internalized and met the prevailing standards for appearance. But as she learned to listen to her body, she had to abandon those standards. Uncontainable sickness forced adopting other priorities for her body. Like this woman, other people cease to measure their body against past perfection, or past hopes of perfecting it, and begin to live with it. The sick body becomes familiar and perhaps even comfortable. This familiarity and comfort increases if treatments, regimens, or health practices seem to work. If so, the sick body becomes predictable and manageable. The ill person may feel that he or she is beginning to unify the altered body and the self. Arthur Frank (1991, p. 87) identifies this unity of body and self, "As soon as cancer happened to me, not just to anyone, it ceased to be random. I am a bodily process, but I am also a consciousness, with a will and a history and a capacity to focus my thoughts and energies. The bodily process and the consciousness do not oppose each other; what illness teaches is their unity."

Typically, however, this unity has limits, albeit unstated, taken-for-granted limits. Ill people often believe that they have already suffered beyond tolerable limits. Thus, they see themselves as having filled their quota of human misery and earned their right to a just reprieve. They often said, "I've paid my dues [of suffering]." If so, then new, foreboding symptoms or conditions shock them. Moreover, these people experience the unpredictability of their bodies afresh as they grapple with new or intensified distress. Their uncertain lives and their frail grasp on health again takes center stage. For the past year, a middle-aged woman with multiple sclerosis had fought constant, debilitating infections. She said:

> My body is distressed, and it needs attention, and I'm working very hard to give it that ... I really feel with MS, I have a much better hold on it, handle on the MS, much better visualization where I'll be in—what I'll do with it in five years, ten years, because I can adapt as I go along. The problem with infections is that infections going on with MS can alter the disease severely in a negative way, and so I want to get more of a handle on the infections.

After being diagnosed and experiencing her condition for over fourteen years, having multiple sclerosis with some residual disability had become familiar and manageable. This woman had had several extremely debilitating exacerbations but after each one had improved considerably. For lengthy periods, she struggled with keeping her illness contained by maintaining and protecting her body (cf. Charmaz 1991; Monks and Frankenberg, n.d.). Although she always acknowledged that her MS could take a downhill course at any time, she expected to have ups and downs. The belief that she had faced the worst before and improved, gave her hope and caused her to view her MS as predictable and manageable. The infections, however, posed grave uncertainty. She said, "The aging with the MS really doesn't bother me. Aging with chronic infections—the infections can just screw up your body in so many ways, and so I'm more frightened by that because it's unknown."

The unknowns of the past echo in the uncertainties of the present. Ten years before, this woman's MS symptoms had rapidly worsened. She had said then, "I'm just so frightened … by the unknowns. If I knew that this was the worst, I could deal with that. But not knowing. … My legs are getting weaker and I'm so frightened because of the unknowns. My doctor says I may have to go into a wheelchair. That's my bottom line. I won't go into a chair."

Coping with Changes in Bodily Appearance

Having a visibly altered body provides the experiencing person, as well as family and friends, with immediate images of change. Such changes occur throughout the course of illness. I use the term "appearance" symbolically as well as literally since knowledge of loss can cast new light and force new self-images upon an individual. But not all people with serious chronic illnesses have visible symptoms and disabilities. Looking healthy can undermine a person's credibility with health practitioners. Women particularly have difficulty being taken seriously. One woman who had a recent angioplasty, angina, an old spinal injury, and bowel disease was told by two of her physicians and her pharmacist, "You don't look like you're old enough to have anything like that happen. You don't look like there could be anything wrong." Even those closest to ill people may not understand their conditions and so expect them to function as before. A middle-aged man had an automobile accident while having a heart attack. Although he sustained some injuries, afterwards, he looked healthy and fit. He lost weight, exercised, and his injuries slowly healed. Yet he had residual fatigue, occasional memory loss, emotional swings, and lethargy from his multiple medications. Because he seemed to have regained health, his losses remained masked. Subsequently, his wife lost patience with him as his business declined and he withdrew from the family. She saw him as shirking responsibility.

Relatives and friends may not be able to fathom debilitating changes in a person who shortly before had functioned with extraordinary competence. Youth and beauty render an invisible illness even more invisible.

While in her early thirties, a woman's youth disguised her debilitating arthritis. Her much older boyfriend saw her as healthy and beautiful. For years, her constant complaints of pain mystified him. She could not enforce her identity claims as ill as long as she appeared healthy, pretty, and able. Because of her appearance, both her private and public identities belied how she defined her self. She said:

> I may look like I'm healthy and all this stuff and I get—all these guys start making catcalls and I'm in pain and it just seems incongruous. I go, "What are they whistling at?" I usually identify with how I *feel,* even though I go through a lot of effort to make myself look good, I still identify with how I feel. It's like being—feeling like an old person in a young person. ... It's like only an old person is entitled to have all this pain.

By four years later, this woman's disabilities had become apparent. Although she had long identified herself as in pain and disabled, she also had been accustomed to other people noting only her beauty. Being socially identified as disabled undermined her self-worth and sense of wholeness. She said:

> I think it's real embarrassing. You know, like say if someone can see that I can't walk or something, I'm all stooped over, you know, I catch a glimpse of myself in ah, like a window, it's very shocking sometimes what I see. [I asked, "In which way?" She said:] Well, I can see that, other people can see is that, you know, my leg, I can hardly walk on it. And I feel like somehow I'm not a whole person and ... people can look at it and feel sympathetic, but they can look at you and see you as less than whole, you know. (Charmaz 1991, p. 111)

She added, "Somehow it's almost like a defect to me. And ... , it's frightening, I guess." Five years later her disability was quite marked. Because she questioned whether she still was attractive to men, she had several affairs, which she regretted.

Ill people may evince few problems about impairment or loss of function until a hidden loss becomes visible. For example, impotency can be a problem known only to a man's wife unless the marriage dissolves. The tension between invisible disability and visible impairment becomes evident. Lesley Fallowfield and Andrew Clark (1991, p. 66) show how some British women with mastectomies rejected their altered bodies when their breast amputation was visible:

Interviewer: Can you tell me how you felt about your appearance since your operation?

Patient: Mm, that depends—I think I look OK when I'm wearing my false one, don't you? I don't think anyone could tell.

Interviewer: And without your clothes?

Patient: That's rather different—I tend not to look at myself—it upsets me that I don't look like a woman anymore.

Interviewer: What about when you're with your husband?

Patient: Oh, I don't let him see me, oh no. I couldn't. He'd be horrified. I always undress in the bathroom now.

Like the woman above, other ill people tried to reduce the effects of visible disability on their pursuits and relationships. And like her, they could then reduce the effects of it on themselves and their social identities. One man on kidney dialysis always wore long sleeves and usually a jacket to hide his dialysis shunt. Feelings about visible disability influenced both men's and women's identity goals. When men could not hide or minimize their changed appearance, they often withdrew. Hence, their identity goals plummeted. Women withdrew less but dwelt upon appearance issues in the interviews much more than men. They tried to manage their appearance to handle their feelings and to bolster their confidence. Nancy Dyson, who had a mastectomy, said:

Wearing bright colors and makeup and pulling myself together before I go out is a way of protecting my vulnerability so people don't make assumptions. It's like camouflage. It's sort of like the camouflage is the door and I can open it or not. It is another way of having control over my disease. I choose whom I share my vulnerability with. (Donnally 1991, p. D5)

Women under fifty evinced much concern about the effects of illness on their appearance. I asked a forty-one-year-old woman with lupus erythematosus if her thoughts about her appearance had changed at all in the last five years. She replied with fervor, "I hate my body; I hate my body. Mostly because I've gained so much weight and—and then my face breaks out [lupus has a characteristic rash]. People look at you like something's wrong [with your character]. I don't hate it because it's sick; I hate it because it's ugly . . . . You're supposed to be skinny and pretty."

When changes in appearance are sudden and visible, women may define those changes as tests of their love relationships. A forty-two-year-old woman suffered a devastating reoccurrence of mixed connective tissue disease when she was pregnant three years ago. She had not had such a serious episode for eighteen years, long before she had met her husband. During that previous episode, her boyfriend had left her and her parents had ignored her. She described herself and her concerns during this second flare-up:

> Oh, I was just a disheveled lump, I mean I was a disheveled lump. I'm sort of still a disheveled lump, I feel like in a lot of ways. But it doesn't much matter to me. Yeah, I mean I think in some ways this was a little bit of a test of me with Bob [husband]. It's like, "Here's the worst I can possibly be," you know; "I'm sick; I'm vomiting; I look like crap." And then I gained so much weight, so it's like, "Here's the worst I can be. Are you going to leave me now?" you know. "Are you going leave now? When are you going to leave? Are you going to leave next week?"

Changing Identity Goals
Bodily Changes and Identity Goals

Bodily changes prompt changing identity goals. Upward changes allow ill people to entertain possibilities and try new ventures. A successful transplant, cardiac rehabilitation program, or medical regimen means feeling better and more able. Then people reentered the worlds they left or embarked on new pursuits. They readily moved on with their lives when they had alternatives and when their identity goals throughout illness had assumed moving beyond it. Thus, these people returned to work, or if working, increased their work hours, pursued sports and hobbies, and planned to redirect their lives. Men returned to their careers. A few women started new businesses. Several men and women went back to school.

Bodily changes, including noticeable improvement, do not automatically result in changed identity goals. Emotions and social relationships influence choices and actions. When fear of failure or further sickness permeates ill people's thoughts, they proceed slowly in forming or changing their identity goals. A young married woman who had had cancer feared a recurrence. She resisted investing herself in a valued pursuit because she could not tolerate the possibility of losing it. Her husband's income allowed her to experiment with college courses and low-paying, part-time jobs. Relying solely on self led some people to measure their options, situations, and bodies carefully when they prized their autonomy. These people could not risk becoming immobilized. Paradoxically, they risked becoming social captives of their sick bodies.[4] Under these conditions, people made changes very slowly and avoided taking risks. They often needed substantial encouragement to reach for more challenging identity goals. After spells of sickness, they had difficulty imagining themselves going beyond their current situations. For example, a woman who had lupus erythematosus had wanted just to be able to work enough to remain self-supporting. Her appalling encounters with eligibility workers and social service employees resulted in her avowals never to depend on public assistance. She recounted:

> I didn't think—didn't have any wide horizons. My friend Ken, he told me last year, "Bonnie, I just can see you managing a business," right? I said, "Oh, give me a break," you know. And he even probably said it to me in February. "You know, Bonnie, you ought to open an office and blah, blah, blah." I said, "Don't even talk about it; I'm not interested in it." But it just happened. One day I had too much work and I said, "Wait a minute." So I got up, called the *Times* [local paper] and as I was walking away from the phone, I went, "What did I do?" That's the way it all happened. And my friends gave me [money] to get started in my business.

In contrast, a downward spiral, or sudden serious episode can force lowering identity goals. Ill people must either adapt because they cannot handle the lives they had—even in the recent past—or they realize that they now have a tenuous hold on managing their lives. How do they do it? What social context affects their choices?

Certainly, markedly altered bodily functioning and feeling can undermine present identities or force lowering identity goals (see, for example, Albrecht 1992; Dahlberg and Jaffe 1977; Pitzele 1985; Plough 1986). People with chronic illnesses resist lowering their goals if they believe others need them to function as before. They put their bodies and their lives at risk when they view their identity losses as too great or when they remain unaware of the extent of their physical losses. For example, several heart patients abandoned their diets and regimens after a few months because they no longer felt sick. In addition, people who recognize but cannot account for their reduced capacities tenaciously try to function. One middle-aged woman said, "It was scary at times. I didn't know what was wrong. [I was] not feeling well, and always having to push, push, push. Always behind the eight ball, always tired, always pushing against this wall of fatigue. And trying to keep up, you know."

The Social Context of Changing Identity Goals

Identities bring commitments and responsibilities. In turn, how individuals define these commitments and responsibilities in relation to other people deeply affects their identity decisions. Changing identity goals then takes into account (1) the individual's definitions, (2) significant others' views and wishes, and (3) the interactions and negotiations among them. Once chronically ill people have altered their lives to accommodate to limited identity goals, it takes substantial support to move beyond them.[5] Given their definitions, ill people may only relinquish their identities and their accompanying identity goals when forced to do so. They may develop intricate strategies to preserve their identity goals. For years after having been immobilized by illness, a single woman had balanced her work productivity with her energy limits. When necessary, she simply took time off from work to avoid a full-blown exacerbation or to regain her energy. By carefully monitoring and maintaining her body, she could realize her overriding identity goal of remaining independent. But keeping bodily needs and identity goals in balance can prove to be arduous. Now married, this woman has two young children as well as farm animals to care for in addition to a part-time university teaching job seventy miles away. Her identities as mother, wife, and teacher supersede any illness identity and cause her to persevere beyond her bodily limits. Her children need her; she and her husband committed themselves to not using child care. The family's need for her income also tugs at her, especially since her husband lost his main job. Thus, by realizing her identities, she risks being forced to relinquish them. She compared how she handled illness when she was single with her current situation, "Going through that whole period in my life when I was real sick, I got very used to just listening to my body and how it's feeling and totally going how—by how I was feeling from day to day. And I can't really, I can't always do that now. There's sometimes when I have to push it much more than I would have before."

Before her marriage, this woman was a successful independent entrepreneur. Her autonomy combined with her control over employees' work assignments permitted her to take time-outs from work to nurture her body. More frequently, middle-class and professional men, not women, can fit their work around their bodily needs. When they can control the social context of work, they can realize and further their identity goals concerning it.

A major part of the social context revolves around spouses or partners. In long-term marriages among older couples, loyalty and attachment typically remain unquestioned although spouses may have sharp differences about health monitoring (cf. Johnson 1985). Wives of all ages willingly saw their husbands through crises, even when marriages were shaky. Problems generally arose later as the long-term effects of illness emerged. In contrast, support from husbands and boyfriends of middle-aged and younger women was more tentative throughout illness. These men did not take over tasks as readily as wives did, and they abandoned their relationships emotionally, if not completely, more quickly than women. Women with illnesses sometimes relied on adult children, friends, and health-care workers for emotional support and practical assistance.

Multiple crises and disabilities that cut into pivotal roles (e.g. breadwinner, sex partner) undermined middle-aged and younger spouses' support. Previously conflicted marriages may break at this point. Subsequently, taken-for-granted identities as companion and parent may also dissolve. Conflicts about identity goals may develop in strong relationships. The type of identity goal and rate and intensity with which the sick person pursues it can all become points of contention (see also Peyrot, McMurry, and Hedges 1988; Speedling 1982). A woman with multiple sclerosis wants to do volunteer work in a busy hospital; her husband feels her body cannot handle the stress. A man with heart disease waits for his health to improve; his wife believes that he is becoming an invalid and should go back to work.

Certainly age, gender, work, and marital status shape, but do not determine, the context in which chronically ill adults change identity goals. As Alan Radley (1989) states, what people with chronic illnesses adjust *with* is as important as what they adjust *to*. Their ways of changing identity goals and adapting to the changes also reflect the content of their lives and the meanings they attribute to their ongoing interactions. Money and help make an enormous difference as to how, when, and why people will or will not lower their identity goals. Single mothers often sacrificed their health for sustaining their identities as workers and parents. Money and help also affect how people feel about changing identity goals (see, for example, Albrecht 1992). Possessing sufficient funds allows older men and women to retire early, a socially acceptable disengagement for the affluent. Having financially secure spouses permits others to leave their jobs or to reduce their work hours. In short, money and help allow ill people more choices about which identity trade-offs to make and when to make them.

The social context of changing identity goals may itself change. The designated "patient," financial resources, and potential help may change and thus result in shifting identity goals. For example, one older woman with a mild heart condition felt forced to seek employment when her husband's health declined (after two heart attacks and bypass surgery) and he lost his job (and his pension) three years before his expected retirement. Two years later, however, she suffered a small stroke. Though she had little lasting impairment, she took the stroke as a warning that she had been under too much pressure. She then became the designated patient in the family. Fortuitously, her husband had become re-employed and could again support them. The move of an adult daughter back into their area also meant help with household tasks and errands. Subsequently, this woman relinquished her identity goal of being fully employed.

Identity Goals and Identity Trade-offs

Identity goals emerge and change through mediation of subjective and social meanings. Hence, ill people sacrifice some identities in favor of retaining others. Noted anthropologist Robert F. Murphy (1987) suffered from a progressive paralysis. He did not endure the professional and financial devastation common to many adults with disabilities because he could continue to work in a field in which he had already established himself. Nonetheless, he felt pressured to remain a productive scholar to validate his worth and to command his colleagues' respect. He writes about returning to teaching in a wheelchair:

> My overreach beyond the limits of my body was a way of telling the academic world that I was still alive and doing what I always did. And all my feverish activities in both academia and my community were shouts to the world: "Hey it's the same old me inside this body!" These were ways of protecting the identity, for preserving that inner sense of who one is that is an individual's anchor in a transient world. (p. 81)

Feeling devalued results in weighing interactional costs and in balancing necessities against possible identity trade-offs. To the extent that these identity issues are direct and explicit, people will construct explicit identity goals. Murphy's interactions formed an unspoken yet unyielding mirror that reflected the renegotiation of his preferred identities. Because Murphy's strained interactions with acquaintances at work reduced his self-worth, he avoided meetings and receptions. He knew that he could not conduct field research so he became a textbook author. He preserved his sense of self by choosing his activities carefully and by making identity trade-offs. Murphy viewed textbook authorship as a lesser identity than ethnographer but also saw himself as "too old" for ethnographic forays, which mitigated his identity trade-off. As people shift their identity goals laterally or downward, they may relinquish what others view as the more socially valued identity. They feel their losses. They think about their lives. They assess the costs and benefits of relinquishing activities and responsibilities and, therefore, identities. When costs to their bodies and intimate relationships exceed relative gains, they give up valued identities. A middle-aged woman related:

> I'd come home and I was in such pain—you have to work [on the job] seven hours but you put in eight or nine. It's very stressful. But I never succumbed to stress but once or twice. It was doable because I only worked three days a week. ... But Alan [husband] would come home and I'd be on the couch in such pain I couldn't get off, too tired to fix dinner and he was just wonderful. He'd call at work, "Well, what should I bring home tonight?" And some nights I'd cook, but not many. And so I decided, this isn't a way to live. I don't have to work. ... So it was with great regret, and not something I planned, I turned in my resignation. It's the best thing I ever did.

Concurrence from others strengthens the person's belief in having made the right choice. The woman above agreed with former associates' appraisals of her appearance. She recalled, "I went to a wine tasting that we put on a couple weeks ago . . . and some of the Board members were saying, 'Gee, you look so much better. You were all bent over; you looked terrible.' I did look awful. I need more rest; you have to pace yourself."

After making identity trade-offs, people often try to redefine their identity choices in positive ways. Similar to other kinds of decision making, they want to view their choices as sound. At this crucial point, the tension becomes apparent between acknowledging bodily limits and needs and constructing a preferred identity for those who must make significant changes of activity and direction in their lives. In order to handle their lives, they must integrate self and illness without having it consume their self-concepts. Thus, like the woman above, they may, in effect, view identity loss as identity gain. In essence then, people can move up their identity hierarchy while they move down their bodily hierarchy.

By this time, these ill people account and care for their altered bodies while viewing themselves as residing in their bodies but not as wholly defined by them. Part of redefining personal identity depends upon seeing one's self as more than one's body and the illness within it (Charmaz 1991). The woman above defined the place of illness in relation to identity:

> Fibromyalgia does not define who Ellen Thomasen is. It's baggage I've got to carry along. We've all got baggage. Some of it's light and some of it's heavy. And we'd like to check it in a locker awhile. And sometimes you can do that and sometimes you can't but it's not going to stop me from going on a trip. That's the way I feel.

Simultaneously, she recognized her limitations and her need to care for her body while creating her life and facing an uncertain future. She said, "I wonder if I'm going to be able to be active with my grandchildren... I'm wondering—we don't know what the symptoms are going to do, you know. I plan to fight as long as I can. And by fighting—it's an attitudinal thing—it's also resting and doing the things you need to do. I don't—I've always been so active that I don't like this at all. But it's doable, you know?"

Finding the balance between struggling with illness and relinquishing identity goals permits ill people to construct valued lives. A woman with multiple sclerosis once felt deep regrets about lost chances and dashed hopes. She feared then "that having MS will affect my life in a negative way," as well as affect her husband and children seriously. Although ten years later she had relinquished some earlier dreams, she had also realized several, including traveling, which she had expected to forego. Deeply imbedded in her family life, she could now say, "I'm comfortable with who I am, where I am."[6]

Surrendering to the Sick Body

Surrendering means to stop pushing bodily limits, to stop fighting the episode or the entire illness. The quest for control over illness ceases and the flow with the bodily experience increases. Surrender means awareness of one's ill body and a willingness and relief to flow with it (cf. Denzin 1987a; 1987b). A person ceases to struggle against illness and against a failing body at least at this specific time. Through surrendering, the

178

person anchors bodily feelings in self. No longer does he or she ignore, gloss over, or deny these feelings and view the ill body as apart from self.

Conditions for surrender to occur include (1) relinquishing the quest for control over one's body, (2) giving up notions of victory over illness, (3) affirming, however implicitly, that one's self is tied to the sick body. Ill people may surrender and flow with the experience in the present but hope for improvement in the future. Yet they are unlikely to entertain false hopes. At this point, the person views illness as integral to subjective experience and as integrated with self (see also LeMaistre 1985; Monks and Frankenberg n.d.).

Surrendering differs from being overtaken by illness, resigning oneself to it, or giving up (cf. Charmaz 1991; Radley and Green 1987). Being overtaken occurs without choice; surrendering is an active, intentional process. However silently and tacitly, ill people agree to surrender. When surrender is complete, the person experiences a new unity between body and self. Mark Kidel (1988, p. 18) advocates "reclaiming our illnesses as expressions of our own being," to gain authenticity. Like Arthur Frank (1991, p. 1), who views illness as "an opportunity but a dangerous one," Kidel also recognizes that doing so risks opening "ourselves to the full and unpredictable impact of the unknown" (p. 19). Hence, ill people define their experience as newly authentic when they realize that having an ill body is part of them and they allow themselves to experience it. They also may define their past ways of relating to illness as inauthentic. Several people echoed this man's view, "I was just a phony, pretending I didn't have it [kidney failure], trying to do everything everyone else did when my body was telling me I couldn't."

Surrendering also can be distinguished from becoming resigned and losing hope. Becoming resigned means yielding to illness, acquiescing to its force, or to the devalued identities attributed to it. Such resignation means accepting defeat after struggling against illness. When people give up, they lose hope and crumble inward. Passivity, depression, and debility follow. They are overtaken by illness. Under these conditions, people with chronic illnesses can become much more disabled than their physical conditions warrant. They lose interest in their regimens and, perhaps, in living. As they give up, they give in to fear and despair. In contrast, surrender means permitting oneself to let go rather than being overtaken by illness and despair.

Resisting surrender means holding on and, with advanced illness, refusing to die. Fear may propel critically ill people. When they struggle against illness and try to impose order upon it and their lives, they are unlikely to surrender during the midst of crisis. But later, learning to live with residual disability can teach them about surrender. As Arnold Beisser (1988) acknowledges, he learned about surrender through facing defeat. Like many other men, Beisser had earlier believed, then later hoped, that his sustained effort would force change to occur and victory to prevail. Yet no amount of effort changed the fact of his disability. Beisser (1988, pp. 169–170) reflects:

> Defeated on all fronts, I had to learn how to surrender and accept what I had become, what I did not want to be.
>
> Learning to surrender and accept what I had not chosen gave me knowledge of a new kind of change and a new kind of experience which I had not anticipated. It was a paradoxical change.
>
> When I stopped struggling, working to change, and found means of accepting what I had already become, I discovered that that changed me. Rather than feeling disabled and inadequate as I anticipated that I would, I felt whole again. I experienced a sense of well-being and a fullness I had not known before. I felt at one not only with myself but with the universe.
>
> This was not the change that had been wrought by struggle, work and effort, but by learning not to struggle, how to give in, to stand aside and let truth emerge. It was not the tragic truth I expected at all.

For Beisser, surrender meant stripping away the fantasy of recovery, the wish for recovering former wholeness. Still, surrender allowed for being in the flow of the moment rather than wishing and waiting for a mythical future. No longer could pressing symptoms, marked disability, and progressive illness be ignored or redefined. When surrendering, illness merges with subjectivity; it *becomes* subjectivity. Surrendering to illness opens the possibility of transforming the self. By reentering the present anew and flowing with it, ill people gain fresh views of themselves and their situations. External social mandates melt away as the person gains voice from within. Subsequently, a new sense of wholeness of self can emerge. When an individual is very sick, surrender permits unity with the diseased body. Fighting illness at this point may amount to fighting *against* oneself instead of *for* oneself. One woman struggled against Hodgkin's disease for twelve years; she resisted being constrained and defined by her illness. During her last hospitalization for a bone transplant, her last hope of recovery, she realized that her body could handle no more. At that point, she relinquished her struggle and surrendered to illness and death. How do people know when to surrender and to what to surrender? When overtaken by illness, the woman who resisted relinquishing her responsibilities said of surrendering:

> It means that I don't have—I can't control it [ill body] and [it means] to look at what it has to teach me. Just . . . let it tell me what it needs to tell me. You know, that willingness and that acceptance . . . . So it didn't come instantly, but I was willing to surrender and to look at what was going on. But it did come; it did happen. And I'm always much more at peace after I'm able to do that anyway.

Fighting for her meant fighting for control over an unwilling body. Surrender allowed her to find new integration of body and self. She disclosed, "I become more when I surrender, I mean I become more; my spirit's able to grow. And it can't do that if I'm holding on to control."

In this sense, by freeing the self from a quest for control, it becomes possible to experience the moment and to allow the boundaries of self to flow and to expand. Yet self also anchors the person to continuity with past, present, and future. And that anchor itself becomes problematic while surrendering to sickness. Another woman reflected upon this problematic relationship between body and self:

> To me it's [immersion in illness] sort of moving toward spiritual states where you do lose a sense of self and time as a release. I mean, self is a kind of bondage in a way—so it's wonderful—you move toward heaven—to not have that burden. But the other thing, of course, is that we are here. I exist as Jane so Jane comes back and wants to exist. So that's the hellish side. (Charmaz 1991, p. 104)

Conclusion

The process of adapting outlined above offers a window on unity between body and self in illness. Illness presents the possibility of developing new and deeper meanings of the relation between body and self. Such possibilities remain more hidden and implicit in ordinary adult life. But as ill people go through and emerge from crises, complications, and flare-ups, they also reenter mundane adult worlds. Meanings gained through experiencing surrender may fade and recede into the past. Yet these meanings and their accompanying feelings may be reawakened and remembered when illness progresses and health again fails.

Appearance issues affect women more heavily than men. However, compared to men, women show greater resilience in the face of illness and greater ability to adapt and flow with the experience of illness. Men more often than women take an all-or-nothing approach to identity goals. They place a higher stake in recapturing the past and with it, their past identities (cf. Charmaz 1994). If they cannot reclaim all of their past identities, they drop the struggle. Failing to achieve their preferred identities becomes tantamount to complete failure. Under these conditions, such men give up.

How might adapting affect those whose lives are intertwined with an ill person? Whether they welcome adapting or define it as defeat depends on their views and interests. Adapting can cause havoc in the lives of people who depend on the ill person and who cannot or will not renegotiate or relinquish earlier reciprocities. If family and friends believe the proper stance toward illness is struggling against it or politely ignoring it, then they will be displeased to witness their ill person adapting to it. More likely, however, family and friends are relieved when the ill person begins to adapt. As he or she does so, earlier anger, self-pity, guilt, and blame dissipate. Adapting leads to taking responsibility for self. Hence, spouses and partners may feel much less need to monitor the ill person and to patrol his or her activities. Moreover, chronically ill people who adapt do not require their friends and family to construct a fictional present and mythical future with them. Adapting fosters candor and openness. And ultimately, surrendering to illness permits grave illness and death to be a part of life for the survivors as well as the sick person.

Adapting to impairment takes people with serious chronic illness on an odyssey of self (cf. Charmaz 1991). Their bodies become alien terrain. Their altered lives can transport them into unfamiliar worlds where they feel estranged. Furthermore, the familiar becomes strange when altered bodies pose new constraints, require careful scrutiny, and force attending to time, space, movement, and other people in new ways. By struggling with illness while constructing their lives, chronically ill people feel that they regain lost control over their bodies and their lives. By regaining control and coping with bodily changes, these people learn to live with their illnesses. As they do, the strange becomes familiar. Because surrendering to the sick body strips the journey of routine distractions and obstacles, conditions exist for ill persons to experience self anew and to continue the odyssey with renewed clarity and purpose. In this sense then, adapting to impairment fosters redemption and transcendence of self.[7]

Through struggle and surrender, ill people paradoxically grow more resolute in self as they adapt to impairment. They suffer bodily losses but gain themselves. Their odyssey leads them to a deeper level of awareness—of self, of situation, of their place with others. They believe in their inner strength as their bodies crumble. They transcend their bodies as they surrender control. The self is of the body yet beyond it. With this stance comes a sense of resolution and an awareness of timing. Ill people grasp when to struggle and when to flow into surrender. They grow impervious to social meanings, including being devalued. They can face the unknown without fear while remaining themselves. At this point, chronically ill people may find themselves in the ironic position of giving solace and comfort to the healthy. They gain pride in knowing that their selves have been put to test—a test of character, resourcefulness, and will. They know they gave themselves to their struggles and lived their loss with courage.

Yet the odyssey seldom remains a single journey for these chronically ill people. Frequently, they repeat their journey on the same terrain over and over and, also, find themselves transported to unplanned side trips and held captives within hostile territories as they experience setbacks, flare-ups, complications, and secondary conditions. Still they may discover that each part of their odyssey not only poses barriers, but also brings possibilities for resolution and renewal.

Acknowledgments

This article was presented at the annual meetings of the Society for Symbolic Interaction, August 15-16, 1993, in Miami. Thanks are due to members of the Sonoma State University Faculty Writing Group, Julia Allen, Judith Abbott, Ellen Carlton, Pat Jackson, Catherine Nelson, and Margaret Purser, for their reviews of an earlier draft. I also appreciate the thoughtful comments provided by Norman K. Denzin and Lyn H. Lofland. The research was partially supported through a 1993 award from the Mini-grant Program at Sonoma State University. I am grateful to Jennifer Dunn and Jane Ermatinger for their participation in the data collection phase of the project.

Notes

1. I am indebted to Margaret Purser (personal communication, 1993) for the term "continuing metaphors of opposition."
2. Olesen et al. (1990) refer to this type of self-appraisal as the self as knower. They argue that through a hurting body, people view their bodies as significant reference points in relation to self and illness.
3. When someone does not understand the diagnosis and its implications, the possibilities for objectifying the body increase. This process intensifies if the person and those around him or her also have little understanding of chronicity. If so, the person may detach self from his or her impaired body. In any case, illness can be such an assault upon the self that the person views his or her bodily changes as unreal (cf. Manning 1991).
4. Physical loss can consume caregivers as well as their patients. Maggie Strong (1988, p. 254) reveals how her husband's continued physical losses steadily consumed *her* self and body:

   Ted's hearing wasn't improving at all. Was he going to lose hearing next? Stunning, a stunning loss.
   Would I now become his senses, not just his hands and legs and fingers? Stunning, a stunning possibility. . . . My sorrow for Ted's hearing faded into a growing panic and rage. He was climbing right into my body. I was climbing right into his, into his sensory lobes, into his auditory cortex and he into

mine. This was a gradual total body transplant in which my own self would be entirely usurped.

Ian Robinson (1988) invokes Strauss et al.'s (1984) concept of "identity spread" to address similar themes. Robinson quotes the wife of a man who had multiple sclerosis: "At this time [when her husband was badly affected] I felt completely overtaken by MS. I saw it, spoke it, lived it, hated it, all day, everyday. Any outside contact was MS; any visitor was to see Walter and see how his MS was" (p. 57).

5. Formal and informal social support for changing identity is geared more to the young and middle-aged than the old. Thus, younger and middle-aged adults have more access to formal support through rehabilitation counseling and therapy than older people and more incentives and prods from others to reconstruct their lives. As people get older, decisions once set into motion, like retirement, become increasingly difficult to undo. The social structure affords older people fewer alternatives for change.

6. The comfort that chronically ill middle-aged people gain with their bodies and their identities echoes studies in aging that demonstrate greater self-acceptance of professionals in their fifties (Karp 1988; 1992). Similarly, marital and occupational status may greatly affect this self-acceptance. Middle-aged men and women in long-term stable marriages, for example, seemed most self-accepting.

7. I am indebted to Norman K. Denzin (personal communication, 1993) for reminding me of the cultural myth of redemption after loss followed by transcendence of self (see also, Charmaz 1991).

References

Albrecht, Gary. (1992.) The Social Experience of Disability. Pp. 1–18 in *Social Problems*, Edited by Craig Calhoun and George Ritzer. New York: McGraw-Hill.

Beisser, Arnold R. (1988). *Flying without Wings: Personal Reflections on Being Disabled*, New York: Doubleday.

Blumer, Herbert. (1969). *Symbolic Interactionism*. Englewood Cliffs, NJ: Prentice-Hall.

Brody, Howard. (1987). *Stories of Sickness*. New Haven: Yale University Press.

Burke, Peter J. (1980). The Self: Measurements from an Interactionist Perspective. *Social Psychology Quarterly, 43*, 18–29.

Bury, Michael. (1982). Chronic Illness as Biographical Disruption. *Sociology of Health & Illness* 4:167–182.

Bury, Michael (1988). "Meanings at Risk: The Experience of Arthritis." Pp. 89–116 in *Living with Chronic Illness*, edited by Robert Anderson and Michael Bury. London: Unwin Hyman.

Bury, Michael (1991). The Sociology of Chronic Illness: A Review of Research and Prospects. *Sociology of Health & Illness* 13:452–468.

Charmaz, Kathy. (1980). *The Social Reality of Death*. Reading, MA: Addison-Wesley.

Charmaz, Kathy (1983). The Grounded Theory Method: An Explication and Interpretation. Pp. 109–126 in *Contemporary Field Research*, edited by Robert M. Emerson. Boston: Little, Brown.

Charmaz, Kathy. (1987). Struggling for a Self: Identity Levels of the Chronically Ill. Pp. 283–321 in *Research in the Sociology of Health Care: The Experience and Management of Chronic Illness*, Vol. 6, edited by Julius A. Roth and Peter Conrad. Greenwich, CT: JAI Press.

Charmaz, Kathy (1990). Discovering' Chronic Illness: Using Grounded Theory. *Social Science & Medicine, 30*, 1161–1172.

Charmaz, Kathy (1991). *Good Days, Bad Days: The Self in Chronic Illness and Time*. New Brunswick, NJ: Rutgers University Press.

Charmaz, Kathy (1994a). Discoveries of Self in Chronic Illness. Pp. 226–242 in *Doing Everyday Life: Ethnography as Human Lived Experience*, edited by Mary Lorenz Dietz, Robert Prus, and William Shaffir. Mississauga, Ontario: Copp Clark Longman.

Charmaz, Kathy (1994b). Identity dilemmas of chronically ill men. *The Sociological Quarterly* 35(2), 269–288.

Charmaz, Kathy (1995). Learning Grounded Theory. Pp. 27–49 in *Rethinking Psychology:* Vol. 2, *Rethinking Methods in Psychology,* edited by Jonathan Smith, Rom Harré, and Luk Van Langenhove. London: Sage.

Cooley, Charles H. (1902). *Human Nature and Social Order.* New York: Charles Scribner's Sons.

Corbin, Juliet, & Anselm L. Strauss. (1987). "Accompaniments of Chronic Illness: Changes in Body, Self, Biography, and Biographical Time." Pp. 249–281 in *Research in the Sociology of Health Care: The Experience and Management of Chronic Illness,* Vol. 6, edited by Julius A. Roth and Peter Conrad. Greenwich, CT: JAI Press.

Corbin, Juliet, & Anselm L. Strauss (1988). *Unending Work and Care: Managing Chronic Illness at Home.* San Francisco: Jossey-Bass.

Dahlberg, Charles Clay, & Joseph Jaffe. (1977). *Stroke: A Doctor's Personal Story of His Recovery.* New York: Norton.

Dawson, Lorne L., & Robert C. Prus. (1992). Interactionist Ethnography and Postmodernist Discourse: Affinities and Disjunctures in Approaching Human Lived Experience. Paper presented at the Qualitative Research Conference, Carleton University, Ottawa.

Denzin, Norman K. (1987a). *The Alcoholic Self.* Newbury Park, CA: Sage.

Denzin, Norman K. (1987b). *The Recovering Alcoholic.* Newbury Park, CA: Sage.

Denzin, Norman K. (1988). *Interpretive Interactionism.* Newbury Park, CA: Sage.

DiGiacomo, Susan M. (1992). Metaphor as Illness: Postmodern Dilemmas in the Representation of Body, Mind and Disorder. *Medical Anthropology, 14*:109–137.

Dingwall, Robert. (1976) *Aspects of Illness.* Oxford: Martin Robertson.

Donnally, Trish. (1991). Healing Power of Looking Good. *San Francisco Chronicle,* July 10. D3–5.

Fabrega, Horace, Jr., & Peter K. Manning. (1972). "Disease, Illness and Deviant Careers." Pp. 93–116 in *Theoretical Perspectives on Deviance,* Edited by Robert A. Scott & Jack D. Douglas. New York: Basic.

Fallowfield, Lesley with Andrew Clark. (1991). *Breast Cancer.* London: Tavistock.

Fisher, Gregg Charles, with Stephen E. Straus, Paul R. Cheney, and James M. Oleske. (1987). *Chronic Fatigue Syndrome.* New York: Warner Books.

Frank, Arthur W. (1990). Bringing Bodies Back In: A Decade Review. *Theory, Culture & Society* 7, 131–162.

Frank, Arthur W. (1991a). *At the Will of the Body.* Boston: Houghton Mifflin.

Frank, Arthur W. (1991b). For a Sociology of the Body: an Analytical Review. Pp. 36–102 in *The Body: Social Process and Cultural Theory*, Edited by Mike Featherstone, Mike Hepworth, and Bryan S. Turner. London: Sage.

Frankenberg, Ronald. (1990.) Disease, Literature and the Body in the Era of AIDS—A Preliminary Exploration. *Sociology of Health & Illness 12*, 351–360.

Freund, Peter E. S. (1982). *The Civilized Body: Social Domination, Control, and Health*. Philadelphia, PA: Temple University Press.

Freund, Peter E. S. (1988). "Bringing Society into the Body: Understanding Socialized Human Nature." *Theory and Society, 17*, 839–864.

Freund, Peter E. S. (1990). "The Expressive Body: A Common Ground for the Sociology of Emotions and Health and Illness." *Sociology of Health & Illness, 12*, 452–477.

Gadow, Sally. (1982). Body and Self: A Dialectic. Pp. 86–100 in *The Humanity of the Ill: Phenomenological Perspectives*, Edited by Victor Kestenbaum. Knoxville: University of Tennessee Press.

Gerhardt, Uta. (1979). Coping and Social Action: Theoretical Reconstruction of the Life-event Approach. *Sociology of Health & Illness, 1*, 195–225.

Gerhardt, Uta (1989). *Ideas about Illness: An Intellectual and Political History of Medical Sociology*. New York: New York University Press.

Glaser, Barney G. (1978). *Theoretical Sensitivity*. Mill Valley, CA: Sociology Press.

Glaser, Barney G. and Anselm L. Strauss. (1967). *The Discovery of Grounded Theory*. Chicago: Aldine.

Glassner, Barry. (1988). *Bodies*. New York: Putnam.

Glassner, Barry. (1989). Fitness and the Postmodern Self. *Journal of Health and Social Behavior, 30*:180–191.

Goffman, Erving. (1963). *Stigma*. Englewood Cliffs, NJ: Prentice-Hall.

Herzlich, Claudine. (1973). *Health and Illness: A Social Psychological Analysis*. London: Academic Press.

Herzlich, Claudine & Janine Pierret. (1984). *Illness and Self in Society*. Baltimore: Johns Hopkins University Press.

Hewitt, John P. (1992). *Self and Society*. New York: Simon and Schuster.

Johnson, Colleen Leahy. (1985). The Impact of Illness on Late-life Marriages. *Journal of Marriage and the Family 47*, 165–172.

Kahane, Deborah H. (1990). *No Less a Woman*. New York: Prentice-Hall.

Karp, David. (1988). A Decade of Reminders: Changing Age Consciousness Between Fifty and Sixty Years Old. *Gerontologist 28*:727–738.

Karp, David. (1992). Professionals beyond Midlife: Some Observations on Work Satisfaction in the Fifty- to Sixty-Year Decade. Pp. 99–116 in *Aging, Self, and Community: A Collection of Readings,* Edited by Jaber Gubrium and Kathy Charmaz. Greenwich, CT: JAI Press.

Kelly, Michael. (1992) Self, Identity and Radical Surgery. *Sociology of Health & Illness 14,* 390–415.

Kestenbaum, Victor. (1982). Introduction: The Experience of Illness. Pp. 3–38 in *The Humanity of the Ill: Phenomenological Perspectives,* Edited by Victor Kestenbaum. Knoxville: University of Tennessee Press.

Kidel, Mark. (1988). Illness and Meaning. Pp. 4–21 in *The Meaning of Illness,* Edited by Mark Kidel and Susan Rowe-Leete. London: Routledge.

Kotarba, Joseph A. 1983. *Chronic Pain: Its Social Dimensions.* Beverly Hills, CA: Sage.

Kotarba, Joseph A. (1994). Thoughts on the Body: Past, Present, and Future. *Symbolic Interaction 17,* 225–230.

Kubler-Ross, Elisabeth. (1969). *On Death and Dying.* New York: Macmillan.

LeMaistre, Joanne. (1985). *Beyond Rage: The Emotional Impact of Chronic Illness.* Oak Park, IL: Alpine Guild.

Lindesmith, Alfred, Anselm L. Strauss, and Norman K. Denzin. (1988). *Social Psychology.* Englewood Cliffs, NJ: Prentice-Hall.

Locker, David. (1983). *Disability and Disadvantage: The Consequences of Chronic Illness.* London: Tavistock.

Lofland, John, & Lyn H. Lofland. (1994). *Analyzing Social Settings.* Belmont, CA: Wadsworth.

MacDonald, Lea. (1988). The Experience of Stigma: Living with Rectal Cancer. Pp. 177–202 in *Living with Chronic Illness,* Edited by Robert Anderson and Michael Bury. London: Unwin Hyman.

Mairs, Nancy. (1989). *Remembering the Bonehouse: An Erotics of Place and Space.* New York: Harper and Row.

Manning, Peter. K. (1991). The Unreality of the Body. Paper presented at the Stone Symposium of the Society for the Study of Symbolic Interaction, University of California, San Francisco.

Mead, George Herbert. (1934). *Mind, Self and Society.* Chicago: University of Chicago Press.

Monks, Judith, & Ronald Frankenberg. n.d. The Presentation of Self, Body and Time in the Life Stories and Illness Narratives of People with Multiple Sclerosis. Unpublished manuscript, Brunel University.

Murphy, Robert F. (1987). *The Body Silent.* New York: Henry Holt.

Olesen, Virginia. (1994). Problematic Bodies: Past, Present, and Future. *Symbolic Interaction 17*, 231–237.

Olesen, Virginia, Leonard Schatzman, Nellie Droes, Diane Hatton, & Nan Chico. (1990). The Mundane Ailment and the Physical Self: Analysis of the Social Psychology of Health and Illness. *Social Science & Medicine, 30*, 449–455.

Peyrot, Mark, James F. McMurry, Jr., & Richard Hedges. (1988). Marital Adjustment to Adult Diabetes: Interpersonal Congruence and Spouse Satisfaction. *Journal of Marriage and the Family, 50*, 363–376.

Pitzele, Sefra Kobrin. (1985). *We Are Not Alone: Learning to Live with Chronic Illness*. New York: Workman.

Plough, Alonzo L. (1986). *Borrowed Time: Artificial Organs and the Politics of Extending Lives*. Philadelphia: Temple University Press.

Prus, Robert C. (1995). *Symbolic Interaction and Ethnographic Research: Intersubjectivity and the Study of Human Lived Experience*. Albany, NY: State University of New York Press.

Radley, Alan. (1989). Style, Discourse and Constraint in Adjustment to Chronic Illness. *Sociology of Health & Illness, 11*, 230–252.

Radley, Alan. (1991). *The Body and Social Psychology*. New York: Springer-Verlag.

Radley, Alan, & Ruth Green. (1985). Styles of Adjustment to Coronary Graft Surgery. *Social Science & Medicine 20*, 461–472.

Radley, Alan, & Ruth Green. (1987). Illness as Adjustment: A Methodology and Conceptual Framework. *Sociology of Health & Illness, 9*, 179–206.

Register, Cherie. 1(987). *Living with Chronic Illness*. New York: Free Press.

Robinson, Ian. (1988). *Multiple Sclerosis*. London: Tavistock.

Sanders, Clinton R. (1990). *Customizing the Body*. Philadelphia, PA: Temple University Press.

Scheper-Hughes, Nancy, & Margaret M. Lock. (1987). The Mindful Body: A Prolegomenon to Future Work in Medical Anthropology. *Medical Anthropology Quarterly 1*, 6–41.

Seidman, I. E. (1991). *Interviewing as Qualitative Research*. New York: Teachers College Press.

Shilling, Chris. (1993). *The Body and Social Theory*. London: Sage.

Speedling, Edward. (1982). *Heart Attack: The Family Response at Home and in the Hospital*. New York: Tavistock.

Strauss, Anselm L. (1959). *Mirrors and Masks*. Mill Valley, CA: Sociology Press.

Strauss, Anselm L. (1987). *Qualitative Analysis for Social Scientists*. New York: Cambridge University Press.

Strauss, Anselm L., Juliet Corbin, Shizuko Fagerhaugh, Barney G. Glaser, David

Maines, Barbara Suczek, & Carolyn L. Wiener. (1984). *Chronic Illness and the Quality of Life.* 2d Ed. St. Louis: Mosby.

Strauss, Anselm, & Juliet Corbin. (1990). *Basics of Qualitative Research: Grounded Theory Procedures and Techniques.* Newbury Park, CA: Sage.

Strauss, Anselm, & Juliet Corbin (1993). Grounded Theory Methodology: An Overview. Pp. 273–285 in *Handbook of Qualitative Research,* Edited by Norman K. Denzin. Thousand Oaks, CA: Sage.

Strong, Maggie. (1988). *Mainstay: For the Well Spouse of the Chronically Ill.* New York: Penguin.

Turner, Bryan S. (1992). *Regulating Bodies: Essays in Medical Sociology.* London: Routledge.

Weitz, Rose. (1991). *Life with AIDS.* New Brunswick, NJ: Rutgers University Press.

Williams, G. (1984). The Genesis of Chronic Illness: Narrative Reconstruction. *Sociology of Health & Illness, 6,* 175–200.

Williams, R. G. A. (1981a). Logical Analysis as a Qualitative Method I: Themes in Old Age and Chronic Illness. *Sociology of Health and Illness, 3,* 140–164.

Williams, R. G. A. (1981b). Logical Analysis as a Qualitative Method II: Conflict of Ideas and the Topic of Illness. *Sociology of Health and Illness, 3,* 165–187.

Yoshida, Karen K. (1993). Reshaping of Self: A Pendular Reconstruction of Self and Identity among Adults with Traumatic Spinal Cord Injury. *Sociology of Health & Illness, 15,* 217–245.

Zola, Irving K. (1982). *Missing Pieces: A Chronicle of Living with a Disability.* Philadelphia, PA: Temple University Press.

Zola, Irving K. (1991). Bringing our bodies and ourselves back, In: Reflections on a Past, Present, and Future 'Medical Sociology.' *Journal of Health and Social Behavior 32,* 1–16.

Dialogue: Subjectivity in analysis

Jan: Okay I have something to ask. Phyllis, you said that you don't have to have an exact transcript to give the interviewer so my question is: Is the essence ever in the "Ahs" and the "Umhs" or is the essence always in the intent of the words?

Phyllis: Mmm—let's not forget that you are part of the analysis. And even if I have a tape so I could tell exactly what people said, I would be interpreting what they said in a certain way and therefore I wouldn't need their exact words. Remember, my goal is to develop theory. Therefore, although I like women's voices and people love to read the data bits, but you have to get a little bit above the data—so I don't see it as a problem, but then that's me.

Adele: In teaching, I encourage students to do at least *some* transcription. They are tending to do less and less. So the crucial point becomes—even if you are doing the transcribing yourself but especially if not—is to sit down and listen to the tape and annotate the transcription. Go as slowly as you need to go so you really end up with a mediated but remediated or reinterpreted transcript. But at the same time, I don't encourage them to go to the incredible obsessiveness of conversation analysis in terms of those annotations. I think that people go too far—especially for grounded theory.

Barbara: I just wanted to add that I also have found that in listening to the tape and doing my own transcription—which I do some of—it brings back other things other experiences of the interview. So its not just hearing words, but a whole lot of other things come back— what was going on at the time, what emotions were in the air. ...Which is all a pretty important part of what you want to catch.

Kathy: I encourage people to use tape recorders with field research when doing observations because usually you can't take notes—its not polite for one thing! But when you leave, you can take the tape recorder and talk and talk about the emotional aspects—these flow as the words focus your feelings. To me the emotions are important!

But of course it depends on the level and types of theory you're doing. If you're theorizing, how certain things about emotions work—you need the emotions to blend in your theory. I think there's a number of places where your emotional content forms the theory in productive ways. So I encourage you to attend to emotions—be very sensitive to such conditions!

Barbara: It also gets the silence. If you feel an emotion, there's something going on emotionally while the words may be telling you something different. That contrast is quite important in your analysis. Also—maybe it's my own cognitive limitations—but if I don't write something within the first 8 or 10 hours there's this huge decay curve!

Phyllis: How unusual! (laughter)

7. From Grounded Theory to Situational Analysis

What's New? Why? How?

Adele E. Clarke

Introduction[1]

One of the subtitles I considered for this event was, drawing on Simone de Beauvoir ([1959] 2005), "From 'Great Men' to 'Dutiful Daughters.'" We are some but not all of the major players of the second generation of grounded theorists.[2] And it is interesting that all of us here are women and we all studied with the two "great men" of grounded theory (hereafter GTM)—Anselm Strauss and Barney Glaser—the first generation. The world—including academia—has changed a lot over the past forty years since they published *The Discovery of Grounded Theory* (Glaser & Strauss, 1967). The contributors to this volume demonstrate the

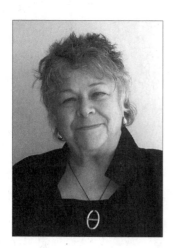

shift from the then predominant "chilly climate in the classroom" for women (if not people of color) to what might be described as "political global warming" fueled by feminism, civil-rights/anti-racism, anti-ageism, anti-war, disability rights, postcolonial theory, and so on. And these changes also inform some of our scholarship.

When Jan Morse extended the invitation to this "GT Bash," I was initially quite anxious. I for one have not enjoyed in the least the tenor of much of the Glaserian/Straussian debate. For some years, Leigh Star (another student of Anselm's) and I took the position of hoping it would "just go away" and intentionally tried not to feed into it. We explicitly did not want to promote the "disciplining" of this or that version of GTM. My anxiety about a GT bash was that it would encourage "bash*ing*" along just such lines. Well, fifteen years after "round 1" (Glaser, 1992), the debates have clearly not gone away, but happily have instead turned into more productive scholarly conversations and have generated clarifications and extensions of grounded theory, including my own.[3] So, instead of aiding and abetting "bash*ing*," this GTM bash is a big gala—a fête. I was reminded of Anselm's comment that symbolic interactionism is a banquet—people come and take what they want and leave the rest (Strauss & Fischer, 1979). So, too, are grounded theory and situational analysis (hereafter SA) (e.g., Clarke, 2003, 2005). I will return to this banquet metaphor.

Continuing to think with Simone de Beauvoir, one is not born a grounded theorist but may, with good fortune, become one. So I will start, a la Strauss, with a bit of intellectual autobiography in terms of how I came to be one and came to be here today. The roots of situational analysis go deep. I was first a sociology student in the scientistic 1960s, at Barnard College of Columbia University (yes where Glaser was, too, though we did not meet then). My exposure to qualitative research there was minimal. But one of my teachers was the esteemed medical sociologist Renee Fox, who was an amazing ethnographer. Another was Mira Komarovsky who, like de Beauvoir, studied gender in the 1950s.

At NYU, where I received a Master's degree in sociology, we were trained only in statistics and survey methods, although many of the faculty did interview-based ethnographic research on the professions. However, Eliot Freidson brought Howie Becker in to give a talk, and we read Goffman, Garfinkle, and other "great men." When I then worked in survey research (for a Columbia University doctoral student), I noticed that some of the most interesting data were left in the file cabinets—answers to "open-ended" questions—because no one knew what to do with them. I had done the interviews and was quite haunted by our failure to include these materials.

A decade later, I sought a doctoral program in sociology that would allow me to specialize in qualitative research, medical sociology, and women's health. I was then teaching in the Women's Studies Program at Sonoma State University, and Kathy Charmaz both directed me to the

University of California, San Francisco (UCSF) and wrote me a letter of recommendation. Her exceptional generosity to me continues to this day.

At UCSF in 1980, I finally "came home" intellectually in all three sites of my desire (Clarke & Star, 1998). As sociology students, we pursued our own hands-on "do-it-yourself" qualitative research projects from design and human subjects approval (yes—even in 1980) to final presentations with superb faculty: Ginnie Olesen and Lenny Schatzman taught field research,[4] while Anselm followed with qualitative analysis organized as a small working group. We were welcome to sit in on his ongoing analysis group as long as we desired. We desired! My cohort also met with Barney Glaser for analysis groups, probably the last to do so as he was no longer at UCSF.

Conceiving Situational Analysis

Significantly for situational analysis, during my graduate studies I fell in love not only with Strauss's grounded theory but also with his social worlds/arenas theory, which he had worked on (individually and collaboratively) at about the same time during the heart of his career. He pursued these as separate projects, more often on his own than with his research team,[5] and his publications rarely engaged both at the same time.[6] But I soon did. Almost all of my own work from the early eighties onward relied on and then began to elaborate social worlds and arenas theory.[7] I was particularly riveted by the idea of social worlds as universes of discourse, bounded by how far they reached in terms of space, time, and meaning-making. Discourse as an analytic concept was just emerging, and I was truly thrilled at having a way to think about and study what we are awash in. I distinctly remember yearning for such a concept in the 1960s.

In the mid-1990s, I began to think about writing about qualitative methods. I was at the time a research fellow at the UC Humanities Research Institute at Irvine in a group focused on "Feminist Epistemologies and Methodologies." Patti Lather (e.g., 1991, 2007; Clarke, Forthcoming c), who became my major interlocutor about methods, was there, too. And this is really where what I later called situational analysis began—from my attempt to reground grounded theory in Straussian social worlds and arenas suffused with the assumptions of feminism that had been part of my life since the early seventies (Clarke, 2006b; Olesen, 2007), and the poststructuralism that had been part of my life since the early nineties (especially Foucault). After I returned to San Francisco in 1996, Anselm and Fran Strauss came to dinner at the end of August, and I told Anselm about my idea. He was excited about this fusion of GTM and social worlds/arenas, and we were to discuss it further. Very very sadly he died on September 6.

What's New in Situational Analysis?

So, drawing deeply but not only on Strauss, SA both extends and goes beyond grounded theory. What is SA about? Why create a new approach? How are Anselm's contributions both preserved and reconfigured for the new millennium? I answer these questions elaborately in my book (Clarke, 2005, pp. xvii–81). I argue for a grounded theory grounded in symbolic interactionist sociology, very much à la Strauss, to be understood as a "theory/methods package." This concept of theory/methods packages focuses on the integral—and ultimately nonfungible—aspects of ontology and epistemology. What can be known and how we can know are inseparable. Such packages thus include epistemological and ontological assumptions, along with concrete practices through which social scientists go about their work, including relating to/with one another and with the various nonhuman entities involved in the situation.

A symbolic interactionist grounded theory/situational analysis theory/methods package, then, is about the "goodness of fit" between the fundamentals of symbolic interactionist theory (e.g., Blumer, [1969] 1993; Reynolds & Herman, 2003; Strauss, 1993), constructionist grounded theory (Charmaz, 2000, 2006; Strauss, 1987), and situational analysis including Foucautian discursive formations (Clarke, 2003, 2005) as methodological approaches in terms of questions of ontology and epistemology. The theory/methods package concept does *not* mean that one can opt for two items from column A and two from column B to "tailor" a package. Nor does it mean that one element automatically "comes with" the other as a prefabricated package. Using a "package" takes all the work involved in learning the theory *and* the practices and how to articulate them across time and circumstance (see Clarke 1991, 2005, pp. 2–5, 2006b, 2007; Star, 1989, 1991a, 1991b, 1999, 2007; Star & Strauss, 1998; Strauss & Corbin, 1997). It becomes a way of knowing and doing *together*. The very idea of theory/methods packages assumes that "method, then, is not the servant of theory: method actually grounds theory" (Jenks, 1995, p. 12).

There are a number of ways in which Strauss's interactionist grounded theory/methods package was always already around the postmodern turn and ways that grounded theory was recalcitrant against that turn— the lurking scientisms, positivisms, and realisms that Kathy Charmaz (2000, 2006) has ably detailed. I won't reiterate those here (Clarke, 2005, pp. 11–19, 2007).

I want to focus instead on what is new in situational analysis. What new possibilities does it bring to the grounded theory banquet table—on offer to all? I will discuss four facets: First are the Chicago social ecologies from the early twentieth century that served as the deep tap roots for social worlds/arenas/discourses theory. Second, I take up Foucault, discourse studies, and moving beyond the knowing subject. The third issue takes the nonhuman elements in a situation explicitly into account. Last are the concepts of implicated actors and actants in situations. I then frame the shift from the conditional matrix to the situational matrix and describe the three kinds of maps that constitute SA. I conclude with some peeks at possible futures of SA.

From Chicago Social Ecologies to Social Worlds/ Arenas/Discourses Theory

Early Chicago School sociology focused on communities of different types (e.g., ethnic communities, elite neighborhoods, impoverished slums), distinctive locales (e.g., taxi dancehalls, the stockyards), and signal events of varying temporal durations (e.g., a strike). The sociological task was "to make *the group* the focal center and to build up from its discoveries *in concrete situations*, a knowledge of the whole" (Eubank in Meltzer, Petras, & Reynold, 1975, p. 42, emphases added). But, as Baszanger and Dodier (1997, p. 16) have asserted:

> Compared with the anthropological tradition, the originality of the first works in the Chicago tradition was that they did not necessarily integrate the data collected around a collective whole in terms of a common culture, but *in terms of territory or geographic space*. The problem with which these sociologists were concerned was based on human ecology: interactions of human groups with the natural environment and interactions of human groups in a given geographic milieu. ... The main point here was to make an *inventory of a space* by studying the different communities and activities of

which it is composed, that is, which encounter and confront each other in that space.

These "inventories of space" often took the form of maps (e.g., Fine, 1995; Kurtz, 1984).

Traditional Chicago School studies were undergirded by an areal field model—a "map" of some kind done from "above" such as a city map (e.g., Blumer, 1958; Hughes, 1971, esp. pp. 267, 270; Park, 1952). Most important here, the communities, organizations, kinds of sites, and collectivities represented on such maps were to be explicitly viewed *in relation to the sitings or situations of one another, and within their larger contexts.* Thus, relationality was a featured concern. "The power of the ecological model underlying the traditional Chicago approach lies in the ability to focus now on the niche and now on the ecosystem which defined it" (Dingwall, 1999, p. 217). Leigh Star (1995) has called this "the figure/ground gestalt switch," and analytically it is fundamentally important.

In the 1950s and 1960s, researchers in this tradition continued the study of "social wholes" in new ways, shifting to studies of work, occupations, and professions, moving from local to national and international groups. Geographic boundaries were dropped as necessarily salient, replaced by *shared discourses* as boundary-making and marking. Perhaps most significantly, they increasingly attended to the relationships of those groups to other "social wholes," the *interactions* of collective actors and discourses. (In today's methodological vernacular, many such studies would be termed "multi-sited." [8])

In SA, the root metaphor for grounded theorizing shifts from social process/action to social ecology/situation—grounding the analysis deeply and explicitly in the broader situation of inquiry of the research project. Social worlds theory assumes multiple collective actors—social worlds— in all kinds of negotiations in a broad and often contentious substantive arena. Arenas are focused on matters about which all the involved social worlds and actors care enough to be (1) committed to act, and (2) to produce discourses about arena concerns. Thus, arenas are sites of action *and* discourse. They are discursive sites in often complicated ways. Particular social worlds are constructed in other world's discourses as well as producing their own. But arenas usually endure for some time, and long-standing arenas are typically characterized by multiple, complex, and layered discourses that interpolate and combine old(er) and new(er) elements in on-going, contingent, and inflected practices. Further, because perspectives and commitments differ, arenas are usually sites of contestation and controversy. As such, they are especially good for analyzing heterogeneous perspectives or positions and for analyzing power in action (a lesson from technoscience studies) (e.g., Nelkin, 1995).

Arenas are also especially amenable conceptual frames through which to work at a more meso/organizational level, analyzing *collective* actors (social worlds), their work, and discourses in those arenas. For example, Peter Hall (1997, p. 397) noted: "A view of social organization is offered that emphasizes relations among situations, linkages between consequences and conditions, and networks of collective activity across space and time." Significantly, it is through such frames that symbolic interactionist studies can address more global elements, increasingly important today.[9] But, like the basic social process/action frameworks fundamental to traditional grounded theory, social worlds/arenas/discourses analyses also cannot do everything we want to do analytically, hence my expansion of them into the several forms of situational analysis.

Foucault: Discourse Studies and Moving beyond the "Knowing Subject"

> Interactionism, if it is to thrive and grow, must incorporate elements of poststructural and postmodern theory (e.g., the works of Barthes, Derrida, Foucault, Baudrillard, etc.) into its underlying views of history, culture, and politics.
>
> —Denzin, 1992, p. xvii

Let us turn now to the first new root of situational analysis: Foucault's work on discourse and the importance of moving beyond "the knowing subject." Simon (1996, p. 319) has asserted that the work of Foucault "might be called a postmodern version of middle range theory." Foucault challenged the social sciences by decentering the "knowing subject" (the individual human as agentic social actor) to focus instead on "the social" as constituted through discursive practices and on discourses as constitutive of subjectivities. Foucault (1972) began with the concept of "the order of discourse," asserting that ways of framing and representing, linguistic conventions of meanings and habits of usage together constitute specific discursive fields or terrains. Conceptually, discourses are analytic modes of ordering the chaos of the world. His concept of "discursive practices" described ways of being in the world that could, when historicized, be understood to produce distinctive "discursive formations"—dominant discourses that bind together social injunctions about particular practices (Dreyfus & Rabinow, 1983, p. 59). Dominant discourses are reinforced through extant institutional systems of law, media, medicine, education, and so on—often operating in conjunction. A discourse is effected in disciplining practices, which produce subjects/subjectivities through surveillance, examination, and various technologies of the self—ways of producing ourselves as properly disciplined subjects (e.g., Foucault, 1973, 1975, 1978, 1988). For example, the various institutions of medicine (from hospitals to pharmaceutical companies) and the media (from newspapers to TV and the Internet) together produce "healthscapes"—extensive narrative and visual discourses on health and the responsibilities of citizens to pursue it. We constitute ourselves and are constituted by and through them—the focus of my own current work (Clarke, 2009).

SA goes beyond "the knowing subject," as centered knower and decision-maker to *also* address and analyze salient discourses dwelling within the situation of inquiry. We are all, like it or not, constantly awash in seas of discourses that are constitutive of life itself. SA enrolls Foucault's poststructural approaches to help push grounded theory around the postmodern turn to take these into account. Specifically, situational analysis follows "Foucault's footsteps" (Prior, 1997) into sites of his serious theorizing—historical, narrative/textual, and visual discourses. Grounded theory aided and abetted by situational analysis facilitates such moves.

Taking the Nonhuman Explicitly into Account

In the postmodern, studying action—the analytic center of GTM—is not enough. So, having begun down the discursive path, it quickly becomes obvious that if the human subject is decentered—no longer the analytic everything—"the object is also and always decentered" (Dugdale, 1999, p. 16). Humans are not enough. Fresh methodological attention needs to be paid to *nonhuman objects* in situations—things of all kinds. These may includes cultural objects, technologies, animals, media, nonhuman animate and inanimate pieces of material culture, and the lively discourses that also constitute the situations we study—from cups and saucers to lab animals to TV programs. Some are products of human action (and we can study the production processes); others are construed as "natural" (and we can study how they have been constructed as such).

Many of us actually using grounded theory have taken the nonhuman into account in our substantive research for decades (Clarke & Star, 2003), but we did so without the methodological reflexivity that would make these innovations explicit—adequately visible to others seeking to use grounded theory in such postmodern ways. Things have also had an important place in interactionist history (e.g., McCarthy, 1984, pp. 108–109; Park & Burgess, [1921] 1970). Blumer, drawing deeply on Mead, offered a specific framework on the:

> Nature of Objects. The position of symbolic interactionism is that the "worlds" that exist for human beings and for their groups are composed of "objects" and that these *objects are the product of symbolic interaction.* An object is anything that can be indicated, anything that is pointed to or referred to—a cloud, a book, a legislature, a banker, a religious doctrine, a ghost, and so forth. ([1969] 1993, pp. 10–11, emphasis added)

This explicit constructionist *and* materialist view of the nonhuman has tacitly informed the research of a number of us (Clarke & Star, 2003, 2007).

Let me further clarify and situate the term nonhuman. Over the past several decades, the theoretical importance of things—materialities—has been retheorized in a number of ways through poststructural lenses. Certainly Foucault's (1973) *The Order of Things* raised fresh ways of conceptualizing how "things" order the world. It was through actor-network theory, developed since c1975 especially by Bruno Latour, Michel Callon, John Law, and Madeleine Akrich in the transdisciplinary field of science and technology studies that I first encountered this move (e.g., Latour, 1987, 2005; Law & Hassard, 1999; Law & Mol, 1995). Actor-network theory initiated a much more explicit and full(er) theoretical and methodological status for the nonhuman and explicitly uses that term.[10]

"Nonhuman actants" are not only present as nodes in the actor network in this approach but also have agency. In science and technology studies, such conceptions exploded dualistic notions of a technical core and social superstructure—the separability of humans and machines. Instead, the social and technical together become a "seamless web," co-constructed and mutually embedded (Bijker, Pinch, & Hughes, 1987; Latour, 1987). Woolgar (1991) captured this vividly in research on "how computers configure their users," featuring the agency of the nonhuman in making us do things differently. With laptops or cell phones in place, we become "cyborgs"—cybernetic organisms (Haraway, [1985] 1991a).

This reconceptualization of the nonhuman as not only important but also agentic is deeply provocative and productive. *Adequate analyses of situations being researched must include the nonhuman explicitly and in considerable detail.* "Seeing" the agency of the nonhuman elements present in the situation disrupts the taken-for-granted, creating Meadian (e.g., [1927] 1964) moments of conceptual rupture through which we can see the world afresh. For example, "Magazines exist to sell readers to advertisers" ruptures the taken-for-granted and offers a different perspective. The agency of magazines per se in the distribution of advertising discourses, normally invisible or at least not the lead point is here rendered explicit and primary.

Significantly, including the nonhuman as agentic actors/actants in research takes up the postmodern challenge of posthumanism—the idea that only humans "really" matter or "matter most." "By acknowledging nonhumans as components and determinants of the arrangements that encompass people, this line of research *problematizes the social and challenges traditional renderings of it as relations between people*" (Schatzki, Cetina, & von Savigny, 2001, p. 11, emphasis added). A key argument in science and technology studies has been that the nonhuman and the human are co-constitutive—together constitute the world *and each other.* Similar arguments have also been made in material culture studies: "Material forms were often of significance precisely because being disregarded as trivial, they were often a key unchallenged mechanism for social reproduction and ideological dominance. ...[S]ocial worlds were as much constituted by materiality as the other way around" (Miller, 1998, p. 3; see also Hodder, 2000). Consumption studies—focused on relations between humans and things—is another site where taking the nonhuman seriously has occurred (e.g., Applbaum, 2004; Hearn & Roseneil, 1999).

Such processes of co-construction and co-constitution can be studied through using the situation as the locus of analysis explicitly including all analytically pertinent nonhuman (including technical) elements along with the human in situational maps. This is one of the key ways in which a GTM rooted in symbolic interactionism offers a distinctively *materialist* constructionism through SA. Nonhuman actants structurally condition the interactions within the situation through their specific material properties and requirements.[11] Their agency is everywhere. SA explicitly takes the nonhuman elements in the situation of inquiry into account both materially and discursively.

Implicated Actors and Actants

There can also be *implicated actors and/or actants* in social worlds and arenas (Clarke, 2005, pp. 46–48; Clarke & Montini, 1993). This concept provides a means of analyzing the situatedness of less powerful actors and the consequences of others' actions for them and raises issues of discursive constructions of actors and of nonhuman actants. There are at least two kinds of implicated actors. First are those implicated actors who are physically present but generally silenced/ignored/invisibled by those in power in the social world or arena. Second are those implicated actors *not* physically present in a given social world but solely discursively constructed by others in the situation. They are conceived, represented, and perhaps targeted by the work of those others, hence they are *discursively* present.

Neither category of implicated actors is actively involved in the actual negotiations of self-representation in the social world or arena, nor are their thoughts or opinions or identities explored or sought out by other actors through any openly empirical mode of inquiry (such as by asking them questions). They are neither invited by those in greater power to participate nor to represent themselves on their own terms. If physically present, their perceptions are largely ignored and/or silenced. The difference between the two types turns on the issue of their physical presence.

Let me give examples. First, those actors present but silenced/invisibled in the situation of inquiry can be exemplified by women scholars and scholars of color in traditional histories of academic disciplines and professions. They were there in those worlds, doing many things, but their presence and contributions have been largely ignored and/or erased, requiring usually feminist and anti-racist archaeologies to excavate, resurrect, and resituate them (e.g., Deegan, 1990; DuBois, 1993). Second, an example of actors solely discursively constructed are women users of most contraceptives by the reproductive scientists who designed them (Clarke, 1998, 2000), who were rather surprised at women's objections and rejections of the technologies (e.g., Bruce, 1987).

There can, of course, also be *implicated actants*—implicated nonhuman actors—in situations of concern.[12] Like humans, implicated actants can be physically *and/or* discursively present in the situation of inquiry.

That is, human actors (individually and/or collectively as social worlds) routinely discursively construct nonhuman actants from those human actors' own perspectives. The analytic question here is who is discursively constructing what, and how and why are they doing so? For example, a heterogeneously constructed implicated actant is the male (birth control) pill. Most people, if they have heard of it at all, will have done so in the question: "Whatever happened to the male pill?" Nelly Oudshoorn's (2003) *The Male Pill: A Biography of a Technology in the Making* answers that question. Though technically feasible since the 1970s, the very intensity of the discursive constructions of the male pill and of men as consumers of it has delayed its release for decades.

The concept of implicated actors and actants can be particularly useful in the explicit analysis of power in social worlds and arenas. Such analyses are both complicated and enhanced by the fact that there are generally *multiple* discursive constructions circulating of both the human and nonhuman actors in any given situation. Analyzing power involves analyzing whose constructions of whom/what exist? Which are taken as "the real" constructions—or the ones that "matter" most in the situation by the various participants? Which are contested? Whose are ignored? By whom? What happens when heretofore silent/silenced implicated actors suddenly open their mouths and speak? Through understanding the discursive constructions of implicated actors and actants, analysts can grasp a lot about the social worlds and the arena in which they are active and some of the consequences of those actions for the less powerful.

In sum, the tap roots of SA lie in Chicago School ethnographies and pragmatist philosophy. The new roots include Foucauldian discourse studies going beyond "the knowing subject," taking the nonhuman explicitly into account, and implicated actors and actants. These come together in the shift to situations per se as focal—as units of analysis—to which we next turn.

From the Conditional Matrix to Situational Maps

In his later work, Strauss was relentlessly sociological in seeking to incorporate and integrate analyses of structural process in new ways. The term "structural process" was used in *The Discovery of Grounded Theory*:

> One of the central issues in sociological theory is the relationship of structure to process. ... Sociological theory ordinarily does not

> join structure and process so tightly as our notion of "structural process" does. … A major implication of our book is that structure and process are related more complexly (and more interestingly) than is commonly conceived. (Glaser & Strauss, 1967, pp. 239–242)

Thus, from the outset, grounded theory was aimed at what today might be called "deconstructing" and complicating this age-old, tired if not exhausted, binary (e.g., Hildenbrand, 2007).

Strauss pursued this through the methodological framework of the conditional matrix developed with Julie Corbin. And it was most especially through dealing with the matrices, through my own teaching of qualitative research methods, and through my own engagement with science and technology studies that I ended up developing situational analysis.

Through the conditional matrix, Strauss sought to develop ways to do grounded theory analysis that included *specifying structural conditions*—literally making them visible in the analysis. Strauss's interactionist sociology was already rooted in process—classic GTM "basic social processes." He was interested most of all in understanding *action as situated activity* (see Figure 7.1 [Strauss & Corbin, 1990, p. 163]). Note that action is in the center of the diagram—the GTM basic social process.

The several versions of the conditional and conditional/consequential matrices that Strauss and Corbin produced were intended to provide systematic paths for grounded theorists to follow in order to facilitate specifying the salient structural conditions that obtained for the phenomenon under study. These conditional matrices frame a number of concerns that are to be considered by the analyst, generally organized into "levels": international (economic, cultural, religious, scientific, and environmental issues); national (political, governmental, cultural, economic, gender, age, ethnicity, race, particular national issues, etc.); and, depending on where the research is undertaken, community, organizational, institutional, or local group and individual/(inter)actional setting. At the core for Strauss is action—both strategic and routine (see also Clarke, 2008a, Forthcoming a; Strauss, 1993).

Looking at the 1998 *Basics* matrix in Figure 7.2 (Strauss & Corbin, 1998, p. 184), we can see that the concentric circles apparently represent the more structural conditions *within* which the focus of analysis dwells. The structural conditions are portrayed as *context*, arrayed *around* the central focus from local to global (from near the center/core to far away

Figure 7.1: Strauss and Corbin's 1990 Conditional Matrix
(From Strauss and Corbin [1990] Basics of Qualitative Research. Copyright 1990 by Sage Publications Inc. Reprinted with permission of the publisher.)

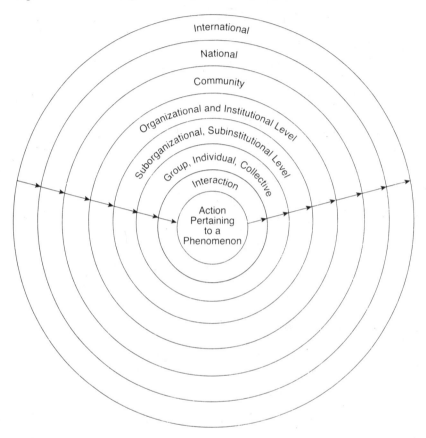

places on the periphery). In Corbin's revisions after Strauss's death, the individual replaces action as the central analytic. All in all, especially given the primacy of the nation state, it remains a very modernist vision. Peter Hall's (1997) critique on this point, which I share, is that "the imagery of the conditional matrix as a set of concentric circles, while perhaps simply a heuristic device, conveys an erroneous vision of social topography, *one that I would rather leave to empirical examination*" (p. 401, emphasis added).

To me, the conditional matrices do not do the conceptual analytic work Strauss wanted done in terms of grounded theory method. Strauss was gesturing too abstractly toward the possible salience of the structural elements of situations rather than insisting on their concrete and detailed *empirical* specification and clear explication as a requisite part of grounded theory *analysis*. Figure 7.3 is my alternative—the situational matrix.

Here *the conditions of the situation are in the situation.* There is no such thing as "context." The conditional elements of the situation need to be specified in the analysis of the situation itself as *they are constitutive of it,* not merely surrounding it or framing it or contributing to it. They *are* it. Regardless of whether some actors might construe them as local or global, internal or external, close-in or far away, or whatever, the fundamental question is: *"How do these conditions appear—make*

Figure 7.2: *Strauss and Corbin's 1998 Conditional Matrix*
(From Strauss and Corbin [1998] Basics of Qualitative Research. Copyright 1998 by Sage Publications Inc. Reprinted with permission of the publisher.)

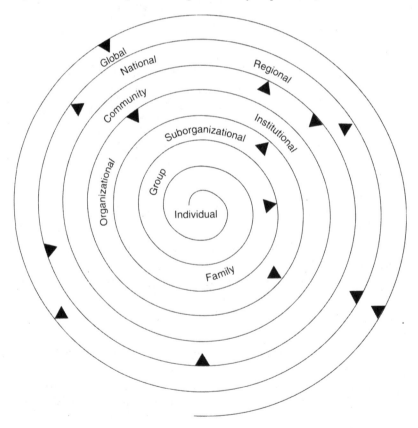

Figure 7.3: Clarke's Situational Matrix

(From Clarke [2005] *Situational Analysis: Grounded Theory After the Postmodern Turn.* Copyright 2005 by Sage Publications, Inc. Reprinted with permission of the publisher.)

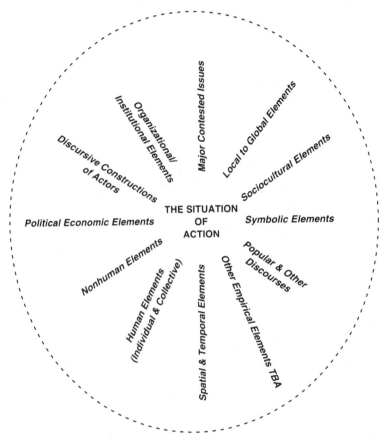

themselves felt as consequential—as integral parts of the empirical situation under examination?" At least some answers to that question can be found through doing situational analyses.

This matrix, like those of Strauss and Corbin, is an abstract version. The diagram as a whole *is* the situation of inquiry. Many kinds or genres of people and things can be in that situation, and the labels are intended as generic. The fundamental assumptions are that everything *in* the situation *both constitutes and affects* most everything else in the situation in some way(s). Everything actually in the situation or understood to be so "conditions the possibilities" (yes, Foucault) of interpretation and action. People and things, humans and nonhumans, fields of practice, discourses, disciplinary and other regimes/formations, symbols, technologies, controversies, organizations and institutions—each and all can be present and mutually consequential.

The concept of situation is key. I was inspired by several scholars here. First, the Thomas's theorem from the 1920s that "if situations are perceived as real, they are real in their consequences," a theorem at the heart of social constructionism and symbolic interactionism, is foundational for SA as well (Thomas & Thomas, [1928] 1970). Second, I was inspired by C. Wright Mills's (1940) work on situated motives, third by Norm Denzin's ([1970] 1989) early efforts at situating research in his book *The Research Act*. And last, a major resource on the concept of situation is Donna Haraway's (1991b) classic feminist theory paper on "situated knowledges" (Clarke, Forthcoming b). The key point is that in SA, *the situation itself becomes the fundamental unit of analysis* (Clarke, 2005, esp. pp. 21–23, 71–73).

Mapping Situations

The situation of inquiry is to be *empirically* constructed through the making of three kinds of maps and following through with analytic work and memos of various kinds.

1. **situational maps** lay out the major human, nonhuman, discursive, and other elements in the research situation of inquiry and provoke analysis of relations among them;

2. **social worlds/arenas maps** lay out the collective actors and the arena(s) of commitment and discourse within which they are engaged in ongoing negotiations—mesolevel interpretations of the situation; and

3. **positional maps** lay out the major positions taken, and *not* taken, in the data vis-à-vis particular axes of difference, concern, and controversy around issues in the situation of inquiry.

All three kinds of maps are intended as analytic exercises, fresh ways into social science data that are especially well suited to contemporary studies from solely interview-based to multi-sited research projects. They are intended as supplemental to traditional grounded theory analyses that center on action. Instead, these maps center on elucidating the key elements, discourses, structures, and conditions of possibility that characterize the situation of inquiry. Thus, situational analysis can deeply situate research projects individually, collectively, social organizationally/institutionally, temporally, geographically, materially, discursively, culturally, symbolically, visually, and historically.

Abstract Situational Maps

In this chapter, I will only introduce situational maps. The initial maps done in SA—situational maps—lay out the major human, nonhuman, discursive, historical, symbolic, cultural, political, and other elements in the research situation of concern and provoke analysis of relations among them. These maps are intended to capture the messy complexities of the situation in their dense relations and permutations. They intentionally work *against* the usual simplifications so characteristic of scientific work (Star 1983) in particularly postmodern ways. See Figure 7.4.

Here I am also going to emphasize something I did not fully realize until I had finished the book—that situational maps are excellent research design tools. Because they are intended to be done and redone multiple times across the life of a research project, there is no one "right" map. If you put something on it that turns out not to be important, you can delete it later or just ignore it. But if it was there in the first place, or got there during the research, at least you integrated it into the research design and sought some data about it systematically and have some sense of its relative importance.

So you can do a situational map to plan a research project. This can be very helpful today in that one typically has to discuss such things even in seeking dissertation grants. The goal for the researcher in doing a situational map for design purposes is to get everything you think might be worth a peek in terms of data gathering onto the map, and then plan what data to gather about it and include theses plans in your preliminary research design. Over time, one adds and deletes from the situational map as your research directions and interests clarify and intensify. If an element falls away, that's fine. Research is *empirical* after all. The map also changes downstream as you pursue what is known in GTM as "theoretical sampling"—seeking fresh data sources pertinent to a particular *theoretical* point you are exploring. Always keep copies of old maps (with dates on them!).

Figure 7.4: Abstract Situational Map: Messy/Working Version

(From Clarke [2005] *Situational Analysis: Grounded Theory After the Postmodern Turn.* Copyright 2005 by Sage Publications, Inc. Reprinted with permission of the publisher.)

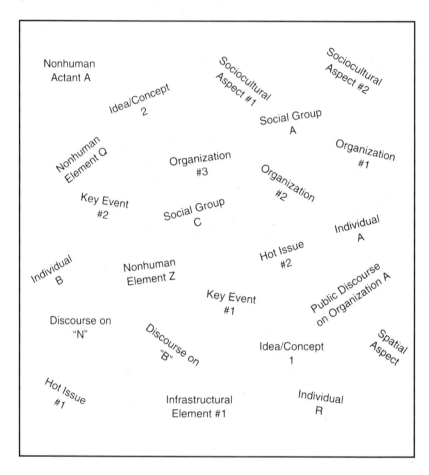

I actually formulated my first situational maps in teaching qualitative research to grad students—usually their pilot dissertation projects. Over the years, I developed the habit of getting one piece of paper going for each student and adding to it during the months of working together on their projects in small groups. As the teacher, I needed a way to remember what they had done already and what we might want to come back to. These messy pieces of paper with notes, tentative analytic diagrams, etc.,

Figure 7.5: Abstract Situational Map: Ordered/Working Version
(From Clarke [2005] *Situational Analysis: Grounded Theory After the Postmodern Turn.* Copyright 2005 by Sage Publications, Inc. Reprinted with permission of the publisher.)

INDIVIDUAL HUMAN ELEMENTS/ACTORS
e.g., key individuals and significant (unorganized) people in the situation

NONHUMAN ELEMENTS/ACTANTS
e.g., technologies; material infrastructures; specialized information and/or knowledges; material "things"

COLLECTIVE HUMAN ELEMENTS/ACTORS
e.g., particular groups; specific organizations

IMPLICATED/SILENT ACTORS/ACTANTS
As found in the situation

DISCURSIVE CONSTRUCTIONS OF INDIVIDUAL AND/OR COLLECTIVE HUMAN ACTORS
As found in the situation

DISCURSIVE CONSTRUCTION OF NONHUMAN ACTANTS
As found in the situation

POLITICAL/ECONOMIC ELEMENTS
e.g., the state; particular industry/ies; local/regional/global orders; political parties; NGOs; politicized issues

SOCIOCULTURAL/SYMBOLIC ELEMENTS
e.g., religion; race; sexuality; gender; ethnicity; nationality; logos; icons; other visual and/or aural symbols

TEMPORAL ELEMENTS
e.g., historical, seasonal, crisis, and/or trajectory aspects

SPATIAL ELEMENTS
e.g., spaces in the situation, geographical aspects, local, regional, national, global spatial issues

MAJOR ISSUES/DEBATES (USUALLY CONTESTED)
As found in the situation; and see positional map

RELATED DISCOURSES (HISTORICAL, NARRATIVE, AND/OR VISUAL)
e.g., normative expectations of actors, actants, and/or other specified elements; moral/ethical elements; mass media and other popular cultural discourses; situation-specific discourses

OTHER KINDS OF ELEMENTS
As found in the situation

---

became inspirational. I realized that it was *not only me* who needed help remembering and holding all the odd pieces together.[13]

See Figure 7.5 for the Abstract Situational Map—Ordered Version. Here you can see the categories a bit more clearly. The categories derive in part from my own work and from Strauss's (1993, p. 252) "general orders" within his negotiated/processual ordering framework: spatial, temporal, technological, work, sentimental, moral, aesthetic, and so on.

In terms of laying out the major elements in situations, these categories seem basic to me.

It is important to note that *there is no absolute need to have all of these categories in any given analysis.* You may also have other categories. Using your own messy map to build this orderly one allows for new and different categories and/or modifications of these. What appears in *your* situational map is based on *your* situation of inquiry—your project. The ordered situational maps should also be done and redone across the career of the research project. Things may well move around. And they may well—and usually do—appear in more than one category. You can learn to do both messy and ordered maps in MS Word.

The key key key key point that I cannot stress too much is that you should not slavishly try and fill in blank categories on the ordered map. I worry very seriously about people doing that. I do so because it would violate the fundamental assumptions of both GTM and SA. GTM and SA are both deeply *empirical* approaches to the study of social life. The very term "grounded theory" means data-grounded theorizing. In the words of Atkinson, Coffey, & Delamont (2003, p. 150): "[G]rounded theory is not a description of a kind of theory. Rather, it represents a general way of generating theory (or, even more generically, a way of having ideas on the basis of empirical research)." The theorizing is generated by tacking back and forth between the nitty-gritty specificities of empirical data and more abstract ways of thinking about them. Philosophically, this tacking back and forth is called "'abductive' reasoning ... a sort of 'third way' between the Scylla of inductive reasoning and the Charybdis of hypothetico deductive logic" (Atkinson, Coffey, & Delamont, 2003, p. 149). "Abduction is to move from a conception of something to a different, possibly more developed or deeper conception of it" (Dey, 2004, p. 91; see also Locke, 2007; Reichertz, 2007; Richardson & Kramer, 2006; Strübing, 2007b).

SA wholly shares in these assumptions. So filling in any "blank" categories of the ordered situational map would be disastrous because it would shift the method from using induction (building from the empirical to the more abstract/conceptual) and abduction (taking back and forth between the empirical and the more abstract/conceptual) into deduction (moving from the abstract/conceptual to the concrete). Yet there is also a tension here that must be acknowledged. The very *doing* of the maps provokes thinking—analysis—and may and should help you work through your data more systematically. So, although blanks should not be "filled

in" mechanically or perfunctorily, nor should one stop thinking and analyzing! If it feels perfunctory, stop.

Note that in doing initial situational maps, the analyst should specify
the nonhuman elements in the situation and how they are constructed
in discourses, thus making pertinent materialities and discourses visible
from the outset. Actually, all three kinds of maps are keyed to taking the
nonhuman—including discourses—in the situation of inquiry seriously.

I use both kinds of maps—messy and orderly—returning again and
again to messy versions precisely because they stay "open" more and more
easily. The ordered ones often seem too final, too fast. Yet my tired brain
sometimes needs the neatness and orderliness to try and make thinking
and writing more coherent.

Exemplar Situational Maps

Next let me provide exemplar maps. I am using as an exemplar here my
project on RU486 (also known as the "French abortion pill") because
abortion politics are so transparent in North America today that I need
not explain much! Approved and used in France since 1982 and in many
other European nations, the contested nature of abortion in the United
States considerably delayed and complicated its approval here. I began
the project in 1989 as an interview/ethnographic endeavor to follow the
FDA approval process "in practice" because it was to have had some local
San Francisco components. Several years later, because FDA approval
was so delayed and the local element had totally disappeared, my third
research assistant on the project and I "ended up" doing a discourse analysis (Clarke & Montini, 1993). RU486 was actually not FDA approved
until September 2000, and even then in a highly overregulated fashion
(Joffe & Weitz, 2003, p. 2353).

The research was not pursued with explicit use of situational analysis but with an incipient form that relied on social worlds/arenas analysis. Analytically, we examined the discursive constructions of RU486
put forward by most of the key social worlds (and some subworlds) that
had committed themselves to action of some kind in the abortion arena
regarding this abortion technology. We focused largely but not exclusively on the United States, and especially on reproductive and other scientists, birth control/population control organizations, pharmaceutical
companies, medical groups, anti-abortion groups, pro-choice groups,

women's health movement organizations, politicians, the U.S. Congress, and the FDA. We also examined what little research existed on women users or consumers of RU486 as a narrative discourse. I conceptualized these women as "implicated actors" (discussed above).

This was a multi-site study with a nonhuman object—a new abortion technology—at the center. Our data included published materials, interviews with key players, documents produced by involved organizations, and observations of some (but not all) key events. [Today, we would use websites as a means of access to pertinent organizational discourses.]

In Figure 7.6, we can see the elements in the messy RU486 map. I have not entered the specific names of the many different organizations involved here, but categorized them under general rubrics (e.g., feminist organizations; women's health movement organizations) for a simpler and more easily readable "teaching" map for this text. Particular organizations would, of course, be entered in the actual situational map and are discussed in the publication (Clarke & Montini, 1993). In the situational map, then, we can see the varied collective actors concerned about abortion, committed to act *and* to producing discourses in that arena. The main nonhuman actant is RU486. Anyone familiar with U.S. abortion politics will note that "all the usual suspects" are gathered here.

Part of the power of SA compared to most other approaches lies in "helping silences to speak"—noting where there are absences as well as presence (Clarke, In prep.). There are two sets of silent scientific collective actors here. Both are concerned with reproductive phenomena and are constituencies for whom abortion is of considerable importance but who seek to keep the proverbial "ten-foot-pole" between their social worlds and the white heat of the current U.S. abortion controversy. First are geneticists and others active in human genomics and/or involved in any and all aspects of prenatal genetic screening. Because there are no therapeutic interventions for most of the conditions current and anticipated screening will find, abortion remains the only therapeutic alternative. Enhanced access to and options for abortion for women who wish to terminate such a pregnancy, such as those provided by RU486, would seemingly be central concerns for these actors. Yet abortion was and remains largely absent from their public discourse. The second silent set of collective scientific actors is fetal tissue researchers—today called "stem cell researchers." They have been silent about abortion despite the use of fetal tissue from induced abortions as materials for certain scientific research.

Figure 7.6: Messy Situational Map: RU486 Discourse Project
(From Clarke [2005] *Situational Analysis: Grounded Theory After the Postmodern Turn.* Copyright 2005 by Sage Publications, Inc. Reprinted with permission of the publisher.)

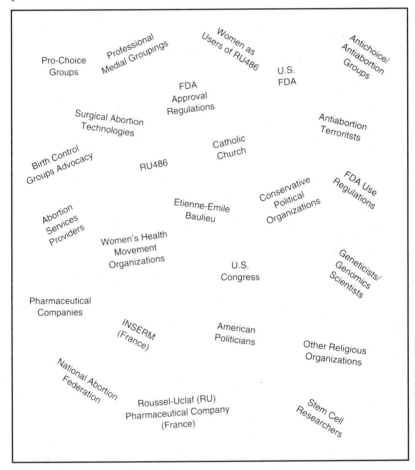

Readers may have noted that I was actually doing situational analyses here. As a feminist researcher, I knew about these silent actors and I put them "on the map"—a map where they would likely rather *not* appear. This illustrates the importance of the analyst's *own* knowledge of the situation in situational analysis as well as the legitimacy of using that knowledge "up front." Specifically, the analyst uses his or her knowledge to help design data collection and does not wait quietly for magically appearing data to speak! That is, the analyst needs to anticipate data that should be

Figure 7.7: Ordered Situational Map: RU486 Discourse Project

(From Clarke [2005] *Situational Analysis: Grounded Theory After the Postmodern Turn.* Copyright 2005 by Sage Publications, Inc. Reprinted with permission of the publisher.)

INDIVIDUAL HUMAN ELEMENTS/ACTORS
Etienne-Emile Baulieu

COLLECTIVE HUMAN ELEMENTS/ACTOR
U.S. FDA
U.S. Congress
Pro-choice groups
Anti-choice/anti-abortion groups
Birth control advocacy groups
Women's health movement groups
Abortion services providers
National Abortion Federation
Professional medical groups

NONHUMAN ELEMENTS/ACTORS
RU486
Surgical abortion technologies
FDA regulations for approval
FDA regulations for use

IMPLICATED/SILENT ACTORS/ACTANTS
Women as users
Genetic/genomic scientists
Stem cell researchers
Anti-abortion terrorists

DISCURSIVE CONSTRUCTION(S) OF HUMAN ACTORS
Social world constructions of others
Social world constructions of Baulieu
Social world construction of FDA

DISCURSIVE CONSTRUCTION OF NONHUMAN ACTANTS
Social world constructions of RU486
Social world construction of abortion
Construction of approval regulations
Construction of use regulations

POLITICAL/ECONOMIC ELEMENTS
Access to abortion
Costs of abortio
Political party concerns re abortion

SOCIOCULTURAL/SYMBOLIC ELEMENTS
Morality of abortion
Morality of unwanted children
Pill for abortion as "magic bullet"

TEMPORAL ELEMENTS
Lateness of approval compared to Europe
Rise of religious right in U.S. politics since 1970s

SPATIAL ELEMENTS
Potential ease of wide geographic availability of RU486
Lack of abortion services in 84% of U.S. counties

MAJOR ISSUES/DEBATES (USUALLY CONTESTED)
Safety of RU486
Safety of abortion
Morality of abortion
Morality of unwanted children

RELATED DISCOURSES (NARRATIVE AND/OR VISUAL)
Abortion discourses
Birth control discourses
Sex/gender/feminism discourses
Sexuality discourses

gathered in the initial design and/or theoretically sample appropriately downstream with great care and sensitivity (Charmaz, 2006).

Figure 7.7 is the ordered RU486 situational map. There are LOTS of discursive constructions because the data I gathered were that. The ordered map reveals one significant individual, Etienne-Emile Baulieu, the scientist primarily responsible for its development and who also served as a public advocate. There were many significant collective actors organized by and large into recognizable social worlds. But the most important new point to emerge through doing the ordered map concerns attending to spatial elements. A key feature of RU486 as a medical abortion technology is that it potentially could be distributed where there are no abortion clinics. Fully 84% of U.S. counties do not have abortion services (Joffe & Weitz, 2003, p. 2354)! Potentially, RU486 could legally put abortion services in the offices of primary care physicians and gynecologists in all of those counties. This element was and continues to be key in the politics of RU486. But as Joffee and Weitz detail, the regulations governing its distribution have limited access to it.

Using Situational Maps to Map Relationality

Relations among the various elements in the situation are key to its analysis. Once you have your messy map, you can do relational analyses. This is the next phase of analytic work to be done with the messy map. The procedure here is to first make a bunch of photocopies of your best version to date of the situational map. Then you take each element in turn and think about it in relation to each other element on the map. Literally center on one element and draw lines between it and the others and *specify the nature of the relationship by describing the nature of that line.* One does this *systematically,* one at a time, from every element on the map to every other. Use as many maps as seem useful to diagram yourself through this analytic exercise. This to me is the major work one does with the situational map once it is constructed. This is one of those sites where being highly systematic in considering data can flip over into the exciting and creative moments of intellectual work. And sometimes there is no payoff.

Relational maps also help the analyst to decide which stories—which relations—to pursue. This is especially helpful in the early stages of research when we tend to feel a bit mystified about where to go and what to memo. A session should produce several relational analyses with the situational maps and several memos. One would return to elaborate on these memos several times as data are collected. They should also be useful guides for theoretical sampling.

Conclusions

SA offers three kinds of maps as fresh analytic devices for grounded theorists. The importance of Strauss's social worlds and arenas theory; Foucault's emphasis on discourse and going beyond the knowing subject; the analytic centrality of the nonhuman; and the concept of situation are clear. I myself am especially fond of "helping silences speak." For both GTM and SA, the theorizing offered downstream in research reports should comfortably "handle" the data at a conceptual level, offer some integration of the concepts generated, be sufficient to address variation and change, and offer a fresh theoretical grasp of the phenomenon that may also open up sites for practical application (on such pragmatist problem-solving, see Strübing, 2007b).

In concluding, I want to look to the future and talk a bit about the emerging generation using and/or writing about situational analysis. Only a few articles other than my own work have appeared to date. Mills et al. (2007, p. 72) supplemented their grounded theory research on Australian rural nurses' experiences of mentoring with situational and social worlds mapping. This generated "increased awareness of how outside actors influenced participants' constructions of mentoring." Positional maps did not work for this project as it focused on action and agency rather than discourses (see also Mills, Francis, & Bonner, 2007, 2008). Polish sociologist Anny Kacperczyk (2007) has published an introduction to SA in Polish. And there are papers in the pipeline of which I am aware. Jennifer Fosket (2004, 2008, In review) has used GTM and SA in her research on a large-scale clinical trial, and has written on the usefulness of doing situational maps. Sara Shostak (2003, 2005; Clarke, 2005, pp. 137–138) used social worlds/arenas maps to plot the disciplinary emergence of toxicogenomics.

Carrie Friese (In review; Clarke, 2005, pp. 139–140) used situational analysis to map the cloning of endangered species in the United States and has challenged the empirical adequacy of the social worlds/arenas metaphor and maps in important ways (Clarke & Friese, 2007). That is, there exist multiple meso-level analytics/metaphors in circulation, and we now think that the choice of which to draw on in a research project should be driven by empirical (rather than prescriptive) considerations. We are therefore considering writing a paper that compares actor network theory, network theories, assemblages, and social worlds/arenas in terms of their empirical strengths and weaknesses. This would update

Clarke's (1991) earlier work comparing social worlds/arenas with other organizational theories.

Last, I return to my theme of being a dutiful daughter. Ans was a brilliant teacher in terms of making you as students do the work of design, data gathering, and analysis yourselves. He was very supportive and asked wonderful questions but would never do the analysis *for* you. As a student, this can be very hard—and disappointing! But the great gift given is that you really learn to do your own research. And that was what he wanted most from his students. I have thought much about being a dutiful daughter, about how to both honor and extend and even go beyond one's revered teacher. Like most of us, I have had much too much academic experience observing those who need to put others down in order to put themselves up. Through working with Ans, I learned that doing one's own work was the best path "up" and that trying to improve tools is a worthy endeavor. I was indeed most fortunate in "finding a creative present in the context of a revered past" (Dunning, 2003, p. 10).

In my efforts to create and sustain SA, I thus felt very reassured by the epigraph from John Dewey on the dedication page of Strauss and Corbin's (1990, 1998) *Basics* books. John Dewey offers a commentary on the importance of change to keeping ideas vital: "If the artist does not perfect new vision in his process of doing, he acts mechanically and repeats some old model fixed like a blueprint in his mind" (Dewey 1934/2005, p. 50). Strauss and Corbin (1994, p. 283) further noted that "no inventor has permanent possession of the invention—certainly not even of its name—and furthermore we would not wish to do so." I hope to eventually become that comfortable about situational analysis!

It *was* a great GTM bash. I hope situational analysis makes useful contributions to the GTM banquet. Please feel free to sample.

Notes

1. Thanks to Kathy Charmaz for ongoing, thoughtful, and useful critique about situational analysis. I have cited fairly lightly here. The complete bibliography for *Situational Analysis* (Clarke, 2005) can be found in downloadable form at www.situationalanalysis.com/

   A current listing of my own methods publications is at the back of this volume. The Anselm Strauss website has his complete CV, topical publications lists, and pdfs of a number of papers, along with a number of essays about his work. See http://sbs.ucsf.edu/medsoc/anselmstrauss (accessed August 27, 2008; see also Clarke, 2008b).

2. In the second generation, in addition to those of us represented in this volume, I would also include (based on publication of their own books on GTM) Dahlgren, Emmelin, and Winkvist (2007), Dey (1999, 2004), Kearney (1998, 1999), Konecki (2000), Locke (1996, 2001), and Strübing (2004, 2007a). Leigh Star (e.g., 1995, 1999) and Antony Bryant (2002, 2006) brought GTM into information and computer science. Kris Koniecke also organized the online journal *Qualitative Sociological Review* (http://www.qualitativesociologyreview.org/ [accessed August 27, 2008]) that features GTM. Thousands of others have, of course, published work using GTM, and there are a number of books on GTM in other languages (see listing elsewhere in this volume).

3. On the diversity of grounded theory, including hollow claims of its use, in addition to this volume, see Bryant and Charmaz (2007, esp. pp. 1–57) and O'Connor, Netting, and Thomas (2008).

4. Their syllabi and reading lists were precious resources and they have been reincarnated annually for the Sociology and Nursing 285a and b courses. The most recent publication of these doctoral-level qualitative syllabi is Clarke et al. (2007).

5. Carolyn Wiener (personal communication, January 3, 2008) responded as follows when I asked her about this recently:

   > We did not emphasize arenas/social worlds in our publications. I was the only one on the team who was interested in pursuing it, stemming from the timing of my dissertation/book, *The Politics of Alcoholism*, which coincided with Anselm's working out the usefulness of this formulation. It fit so beautifully with what I had observed in my first exposure to the alcohol arena at a huge meeting in San Francisco which addressed alcohol problems from a myriad of perspectives. I had been given a fellowship that required I choose a research subject related to alcoholism, which I just assumed was a clearly defined entity. I told Anselm about the contentious discussion in the sessions and described the field as a "mess." You will appreciate his glee when he told me, "That's your subject, the mess!"

6. For Strauss's more theoretical publications focused on social worlds/arenas, see Strauss (1978a, 1978b, 1982a, 1982b, 1984, 1991a, 1991b); for his capstone

statement, see Strauss (1993, pp. 209–244). The only major published empirical study was *Psychiatric Ideologies and Institutions* (Strauss et al., 1964) through which, I would argue, he and colleagues created the framework rather than used it. Wiener and Strauss also wrote an (unpublished) social worlds/arenas analysis of the early years of HIV/AIDS in the San Francisco Bay Area, available online on the Strauss website at http://www.ucsf.edu/anselmstrauss/pdf/socworlds-aids.pdf / (accessed August 27, 2008).

7. See Clarke (1990a, 1990b, 1991, 1998, 2005, pp. 109–117, 2006a), Clarke and Montini (1993), Clarke and Star (2003, 2007), and Clarke and Friese (2007).

8. On multi-sited research, see, for example, Marcus (1998). For examples, see Freidson's (1970, 1975) work on the profession of medicine, and Bucher's (1962, 1988; Bucher & Strauss, 1961) on reform-oriented segments as social movements inside a profession.

9. Other works discussing or using the social worlds/arenas framework include Baszanger (1998a, 1998b), Bucher (1988), Casper (1998a, 1998b), Garrety (1997), Star (1989), Wiener (1981, 1991, 2000), and reviews in Clarke and Star (2003, 2007). Becker (1982) and Shibutani (1955, 1962, 1986, pp. 109–116) also wrote on social worlds, though not using grounded theory methods.

10. For interactionist critiques of actor-network theory, see Star (1991a, b, 1995), Fujimura (1991), and Clarke and Montini (1993). Especially on nonhuman agency, see Casper (1994), Latour (2005), and Law and Hassard (1999).

11. Monica Casper's (1998b, see also 1994) concept of "work objects" generated through her research on fetal surgery nicely allows the question of whether the focus of work is or is not "human" to be empirically addressed. See Clarke (1995), on the salience of nonhumans in scientific research on reproductive physiology, and Haraway (2007), on the vexed boundary between human and nonhuman.

12. Special thanks to Laura Mamo for discussions on this point.

13. As I began to get serious about situational maps, I remembered that earlier, in *Negotiations,* Strauss (1978b, pp. 98–99) had distinguished between a broader structural context and a narrower and more immediate negotiation context. Later, Strauss and Corbin (1990, p. 100) distinguished among causal, intervening, and contextual conditions. This was provocative for my thinking. Although I would agree that some elements are more important than others, and some are certainly experienced by those in the situation as "closer in" than others, it is precisely such an in principle dualism/determinism that I am struggling against.

References

Applbaum, K. (2004). *The marketing era: From professional practice to global provisioning.* New York: Routledge.

Atkinson, P., Coffey, A., & Delamont, S. (2003). *Key themes in qualitative research: Continuities and change.* Walnut Creek, CA: AltaMira.

Baszanger, I. (1998a). *Inventing pain medicine: From the laboratory to the clinic.* New Brunswick, NJ: Rutgers University Press.

Baszanger, I. (1998b). The work sites of an American interactionist: A. L. Strauss (1917–1996). *Symbolic Interaction,* 21(4), 353–378.

Baszanger, I. & Dodier, N. (1997). Ethnography: Relating the part to the whole. In D. Silverman (Ed.), *Qualitative research: Theory, method, and practice* (pp. 8–23). London: Sage.

Becker, H. S. (1982). Art worlds. Berkeley: University of California Press.

Bijker, W., Pinch, T., & Hughes, T. (Eds.). (1987). *The social construction of technical systems: New directions in the sociology and history of technology.* Cambridge, MA: MIT Press.

Blumer, H. (1958). Race prejudice as a sense of group position. *Pacific Sociological Review,* 1(1), 3–8.

Blumer, H. ([1969] 1993). *Symbolic interactionism: Perspective and method.* Berkeley: University of California Press.

Bruce, J. (1987). Users' perspectives on contraceptive technology and delivery systems: Highlighting some feminist issues. *Technology in Society,* 9(3–4), 359–383.

Bryant, A. (2002). Re-grounding grounded theory. *Journal of Information Technology, Theory and Application,* 4(1), 25–42.

Bryant, A. (2006). *Thinking informatically: A new understanding of information, communication and technology.* Lampeter, UK: Edwin Mellen.

Bryant, A. & Charmaz, K. (Eds.). (2007). *Handbook of grounded theory.* London: Sage.

Bucher, R. (1962). Pathology: A study of social movements within a profession. *Social Problems,* 10(1), 40–51.

Bucher, R. (1988). On the natural history of health care occupations. *Work and Occupations,* 15(2), 131–147.

Bucher, R. & Strauss, A. (1961). Professions in process. *American Journal of Sociology,* 66(4), 325–334.

Casper, M. J. (1994). Reframing and grounding nonhuman agency: What makes a fetus an agent? *American Behavioral Scientist,* 37(6), 839–856.

Casper, M. J. (1998a). *The making of the unborn patient: A social anatomy of fetal surgery.* New Brunswick, NJ: Rutgers University Press.

Casper, M. J. (1998b). Negotiations, work objects and the unborn patient: The interactional scaffolding of fetal surgery. *Symbolic Interaction*, 21(4), 379–400.

Charmaz, K. (2000). Grounded theory: Objectivist and constructivist methods. In N. K. Denzin & Y. S. Lincoln (Eds.), *Handbook of qualitative research*, 2nd ed. (pp. 509–536). Thousand Oaks, CA: Sage.

Charmaz, K. (2006). *Constructing grounded theory*. London: Sage.

Clarke, A. E. (1990a). A Social Worlds Research Adventure. The Case of Reproductive Science. In S. Cozzens & T. Gieryn (Eds.) *Theories of science in society* (pp. 15–42). Bloomington: Indiana University Press.

Clarke, A. E. (1990b). Controversy and the Development of American Reproductive Sciences. *Social Problems* 37(1), 18-37.

Clarke, A. E. (1991). Social worlds theory as organizational theory. In D. Maines (Ed.), *Social organization and social process: Essays in honor of Anselm Strauss* (pp. 119–158). Hawthorne, NY: Aldine de Gruyter.

Clarke, A. E. (1995). Research materials and reproductive science in the United States, 1910–1940. In S. L. Star (Ed.), *Ecologies of knowledge: New directions in sociology of science and technology* (pp. 183–219). Albany: State University of New York Press.

Clarke, A. E. (1998). *Disciplining reproduction: Modernity, American life sciences and the "problem of sex."* Berkeley: University of California Press.

Clarke, A. E. (2000). Maverick reproductive scientists and the production of contraceptives c1915–2000. In A. Saetnan, N. Oudshoorn, & M. Kirejczyk (Eds.), *Bodies of technology: Women's involvement with reproductive medicine* (pp. 37–89). Columbus: Ohio State University Press.

Clarke, A. E. (2003). Situational analyses: Grounded theory mapping after the postmodern turn. *Symbolic Interaction*, 26(4), 553–576.

Clarke, A. E. (2005). *Situational analysis: Grounded theory after the postmodern turn*. Thousand Oaks, CA: Sage.

Clarke, A. E. (2006a). Social worlds. In G. Ritzer (Ed.), *The Blackwell encyclopedia of sociology* (pp. 4547–4549). Malden, MA: Blackwell.

Clarke, A. E. (2006b). Feminisms, grounded theory and situational analysis. In S. Hesse-Biber (Ed.), *The handbook of feminist research: Theory and praxis* (pp. 345–370). Thousand Oaks, CA: Sage.

Clarke, A. E. (2007). Grounded theory: Conflicts, debates and situational analysis. In W. Outhwaite & S. P. Turner (Eds.), *Handbook of social science methodology* (pp. 838–885). Thousand Oaks, CA: Sage.

Clarke, A. E. (2008a). Sex/gender and race/ethnicity in the legacy of Anselm Strauss. *Studies in Symbolic Interaction*, 32, 159–176.

Clarke, A. E. (2008b). Anselm L. Strauss. In G. Ritzer (Ed.), *The Blackwell encyclopedia of sociology*. Malden, MA: Blackwell.

Clarke, A. E. (2009). From the rise of medicine to biomedicalization: U.S. health-scapes and iconography c1890–present. To appear in A. E. Clarke, J. Shim, L. Mamo, J. Fosket, & J. Fishman (Eds.), *Biomedicalization: Technoscience and transformations of health and illness in the U.S.* Durham, NC: Duke University Press.

Clarke, A. E. (Forthcoming a). Sex/gender and race/ethnicity in the legacy of Anselm Strauss. To appear in French in D. Chabaud-Rychter, V. Descoutures, A. Devreux, & E. Varikas (Eds.), *Questions de genre aux sciences sociales "normâles."* Paris: La Découverte.

Clarke, A. E. (Forthcoming b). Situational analysis: A Haraway-inspired feminist approach to qualitative research. To appear in S. Ghamari-Tabrizi (Ed.), *Thinking with Donna Haraway.* Cambridge, MA: MIT Press.

Clarke, A. E. Forthcoming c. On *Getting Lost* with Patti Lather. To appear in Special Issue on Knowledge that Matters, *Frontiers: A Journal of Women's Studies.*

Clarke, A. E. In prep. Helping silences speak: The use of positional maps in situational analysis.

Clarke, A. E. & Friese, C. (2007). Situational analysis: Going beyond traditional grounded theory. In A. Bryant & K. Charmaz (Eds.), *Handbook of grounded theory* (pp. 694–743). London: Sage.

Clarke, A. E., Kennedy H., Pinderhughes, H., & Kools, S. (2007). Syllabus for qualitative research and analysis. In J. D. Ballard & V. Jensen (Eds.), *Teaching qualitative methods: A collection of syllabi and instructional materials,* 4th ed. (pp. 79–103). Washington, DC: Teaching Publications of the American Sociological Association. Available online at www.e-noah.net/asa/asashoponlineservice/ProductDetails.aspx?productID=ASAOE339Q07E (accessed August 27, 2008).

Clarke, A. E. & Montini, T. (1993). The many faces of RU486: Tales of situated knowledges and technological contestations. *Science, Technology and Human Values,* 18(1), 42–78.

Clarke, A. E. & Star, S. L. (1998). On coming home and intellectual generosity. Introduction to special issue: New work in the tradition of Anselm L. Strauss. *Symbolic Interaction* 21(4), 341–349.

Clarke, A. E. & Star, S. L. (2003). Symbolic interactionist studies of science, technology and medicine. In L. Reynolds & N. Herman (Eds.), *Handbook of symbolic interactionism* (pp. 539–574). Walnut Creek, CA: AltaMira.

Clarke, A. E. & Star, S. L. (2007). The social worlds/arenas/discourse framework as a theory-methods package. In M. Lynch, O. Amsterdamska, & E. Hackett (Eds.), *The new handbook of science and technology studies* (pp. 113–137). Cambridge, MA: MIT Press.

Dahlgren, L., Emmelin, M., & Winkvist, A. (2007). *Qualitative methodology for international public health.* Umea, Sweden: International School of Public Health, Umea University.

DeBeauvoir, S. ([1959] 2005). *Memoirs of a dutiful daughter.* New York: Harper-Collins Publishers.

Deegan, M. J. (1990). *Jane Addams and the men of the Chicago School: 1892–1918.* New Brunswick, NJ: Transaction Publishers.

Denzin, N. K. ([1970] 1989). *The research act: A theoretical introduction to sociological methods.* Chicago: Aldine.

Denzin, N. K. (1992). *Symbolic interactionism and cultural studies: The politics of interpretation.* Oxford: Basil Blackwell.

Dewey, J. ([1934] 2005). *Art as experience.* New York: Perigee Books.

Dey, I. (1999). *Grounding grounded theory: Guidelines for qualitative inquiry.* San Diego, CA: Academic Press.

Dey, I. (2004). Grounded theory. In C. Seale, G. Gobo, J. F. Gubrium, & D. Silverman (Eds.), *Qualitative research practice* (pp. 80–93). London: Sage.

Dingwall, R. (1999). On the nonnegotiable in sociological life. In B. Glassner & R. Herts (Eds.), *Qualitative sociology and everyday life* (pp. 215–225). Thousand Oaks, CA : Sage.

Dreyfus, H. L. & Rabinow, P. (1983). *Michel Foucault: Beyond structuralism and hermeneutics,* 2nd ed. Chicago: University of Chicago Press.

DuBois, W.E.B. (1993). *W.E.B. Dubois reader.* New York: Scribner.

Dugdale, A. (1999). Materiality: Juggling sameness and difference. In J. Law & J. Hassard (Eds.), *Actor-network theory and after* (pp. 113–135). Oxford, UK: Blackwell Publishers.

Dunning, J. (2003). Limon's troupe now bears her signature. *New York Times,* Sunday, April 27:10AR.

Fine, G. A. (1995). *A second Chicago school?: The development of a postwar American sociology.* Chicago: University of Chicago Press.

Fosket, J. R. (2004). Constructing 'high risk" women: The development and standardization of a breast cancer risk assessment tool. *Science, Technology, and Human Values,* 29(3), 291–323.

Fosket, J. R. (2008). Breast cancer risk as disease: Biomedicalizing risk. To appear in A. E. Clarke, J. Shim, L. Mamo, J. Fosket, & J. Fishman (Eds.), *Biomedicalization: Technoscience and transformations of health and illness in the U.S.* Durham, NC: Duke University Press.

Fosket, J. R. In review. Situating knowledge.

Foucault, M. (1972). *The archeology of knowledge and the discourse on language.* New York: Harper.

Foucault, M. (1973). *The order of things: An archeology of the human sciences.* New York: Vintage/Random House.

Foucault, M. (1975). *The birth of the clinic: An archeology of medical perception.* New York: Vintage/Random House.

Foucault, M. (1978). *The history of sexuality.* Vol. 1: *An introduction.* New York: Vintage Books.

Foucault, M. (1988). Technologies of the self. In L. Martin, H. Gutman, & P. Hutton (Eds.), *Technologies of the self: A seminar with Michel Foucault* (pp. 16–49). Amherst: University of Massachusetts Press.

Freidson, E. (1970). *Profession of medicine: A study of the sociology of applied knowledge.* New York: Harper and Row.

Freidson, E. (1975). *Doctoring together: A study of professional social control.* Chicago: University of Chicago Press.

Friese, C. In review. Model assemblages: Cloned endangered animals as models for biomedical species preservation.

Fujimura, J. H. (1991). On methods, ontologies and representation in the sociology of science: Where do we stand? In D. Maines (Ed.), *Social organization and social process: Essays in honor of Anselm Strauss* (pp. 207–248). Hawthorne, NY: Aldine de Gruyter.

Garrety, K. (1997). Social worlds, actor-networks and controversy: The case of cholesterol, dietary fat and heart disease. *Social Studies of Science, 27*(5), 727–773.

Glaser, B. G. (1992). *Emergence versus forcing: Basics of grounded theory analysis.* Mill Valley, CA: Sociology Press.

Glaser, B. G. & Strauss, A. L. (1967). *The discovery of grounded theory: Strategies for qualitative research.* Chicago: Aldine.

Hall, P. (1997). Meta-power, social organization, and the shaping of social action. *Symbolic Interaction, 20*(4), 39–418.

Haraway, D. ([1985] 1991a). *Simians, cyborgs, and women: The reinvention of nature.* New York: Routledge.

Haraway, D. (1991b). Situated knowledges: The science question in feminism and the privilege of partial perspective. In D. Haraway (Ed.), *Simians, cyborgs, and women: The reinvention of nature* (pp. 183–202). New York: Routledge.

Haraway, D. (2007). *When species meet.* Minneapolis: University of Minnesota Press.

Hearn, J. & Roseneil, S. (Eds.). (1999). *Consuming cultures: Power and resistance.* London: Macmillan.

Hildenbrand, B. (2007). Mediating structure and interaction in grounded theory. In A. Bryant & K. Charmaz (Eds.), *Handbook of grounded theory* (pp. 539–564). London: Sage.

Hodder, I. (2000). The interpretation of documents and material culture. In N. K. Denzin & Y. S. Lincoln (Eds.), *Handbook of qualitative research,* 2nd ed. (pp. 703–715). Thousand Oaks, CA: Sage.

Hughes, E. C. (1971). *The sociological eye.* Chicago: Aldine Atherton.

Jenks, C. (1995). The centrality of the eye in Western culture: An introduction. In C. Jenks (Ed.), *Visual culture* (pp. 1–25). London: Routledge.

Joffe, C. & Weitz, T. A. (2003). Normalizing the exceptional: incorporating the "abortion pill" into mainstream medicine. *Social Science and Medicine, 56*(12), 2353–2366.

Kacperczyk, A. (2007). Badacz i jego poszukiwania w świetle "Analizy Sytua-cyjnej" Adele E. Clarke. Przegląd Socjologii Jakościowej Tom III Numer 2. [*The investigator and his/her explorations in "Situational Analysis" by Adele E. Clarke*]. Available online at www.qualitativesociologyreview.org/PL/Volume4/abstracts_eng.php (accessed August 27, 2008).

Kearney, M. H. (1998). Ready to wear: Discovering grounded formal theory. *Research in Nursing and Health*, 21(2), 179–186.

Kearney, M. H. (1999). *Understanding women's recovery from illness and trauma.* Thousand Oaks, CA: Sage.

Konecki, K. (2000). *Studies in qualitative methodology: Grounded theory* [in Polish]. Warsaw, Poland: PWN.

Kurtz, L. R. (1984). *Evaluating Chicago sociology: A guide to the literature, with an annotated bibliography.* Chicago: University of Chicago Press.

Lather, P. (1991). *Getting smart: Feminist research and pedagogy with/in the postmodern.* New York: Routledge.

Lather, P. (2007). *Getting lost: Feminist efforts toward a double(d) science.* Albany: State University of New York Press.

Latour, B. (1987). *Science in action.* Cambridge, MA: Harvard University Press.

Latour, B. (2005). *Reassembling the social: An introduction to actor-network theory.* Oxford: Oxford University Press.

Law, J. & Hassard, J. (Eds.). (1999). *Actor network theory and after.* Malden, MA: Blackwell.

Law, J. & Mol, A. (1995). Notes on materiality and sociality. *The Sociological Review*, 43(2), 274–294.

Locke, K. (1996). Rewriting the discovery of grounded theory after 25 years? *Journal of Management Inquiry*, 5(1), 239–245.

Locke, K. (2001). *Grounded theory in management research.* Thousand Oaks, CA: Sage.

Locke, K. (2007). Rational control and irrational free-play: Dual-thinking modes as necessary tension in grounded theorizing. In A. Bryant & K. Charmaz (Eds.), *Handbook of grounded theory* (pp. 565–579). London: Sage.

Marcus, G. (1998). *Ethnography through thick and thin.* Princeton, NJ: Princeton University Press.

McCarthy, D. (1984). Towards a sociology of the physical world: George Herbert Mead on physical objects. *Studies in Symbolic Interaction*, 5, 105–121.

Mead, G. H. ([1927] 1964). The objective reality of perspectives. In A. J. Reck (Ed.), *Selected writings of George Herbert Mead* (pp. 306–319). Chicago: University of Chicago Press.

Meltzer, B. N., Petras J. W., & Reynolds, L. T. (1975). *Symbolic interactionism: Genesis, varieties and criticism.* Boston: Routledge and Kegan Paul.

Miller, D. (1998). Why some things matter. In D. Miller (Ed.), *Material cultures: Why some things matter* (pp. 3–21). London: University College of London Press.

Mills, C. W. (1940). Situated actions and vocabularies of motive. *American Sociological Review,* 5(6), 904–913.

Mills, J., Chapman, Y., Bonner, A., & Francis, K. (2007). Grounded theory: A methodological spiral from positivism to postmodernism. *Journal of Advanced Nursing,* 58(1), 72–79.

Mills, J., Francis, K., & Bonner, A. (2007). Live my work: Rural nurses and their multiple perspectives of self. *Journal of Advanced Nursing,* 59(6), 583–590.

Mills, J., Francis, K., & Bonner, A. (2008). Getting to know a stranger-rural nurses' experiences of mentoring: A grounded theory. *International Journal of Nursing Studies,* 45(4), 599–607.

Nelkin, D. (1995). Scientific controversies. In S. Jasanoff, G. E. Markle, J. Petersen, and T. Pinch (Eds.), *Handbook of science & technology studies* (pp. 444–456). Thousand Oaks, CA: Sage.

O'Connor, M. K., Netting, F. E., & Thomas, M. L. (2008). Grounded theory: Managing the challenge for those facing institutional review board oversight. *Qualitative Inquiry,* 14(1), 28–45.

Olesen, V. L. (2007). Feminist qualitative research and grounded theory: Complexities, criticisms and opportunities. In A. Bryant & K. Charmaz (Eds.), *Handbook of grounded theory* (pp. 417–435). London: Sage.

Oudshoorn, N. (2003). *The male pill: A biography of a technology in the making.* Durham, NC: Duke University Press.

Park, R. E. (1952). *Human communities.* Glencoe, IL: Free Press.

Park, R. E. & Burgess, E. W. ([1921] 1970). *Introduction to the science of sociology.* Chicago: University of Chicago.

Prior, L. (1997). Following in Foucault's footsteps: Text and context in qualitative research. In D. Silverman (Ed.), *Qualitative research: Theory, method, practice* (pp. 63–79). London: Sage.

Reichertz, J. (2007). Abduction: The logic of discovery of grounded theory. In A. Bryant & K. Charmaz (Eds.), *Handbook of grounded theory* (pp. 214–228). London: Sage.

Reynolds, L. & Herman, N. (Eds.). (2003). *Handbook of symbolic interactionism.* Walnut Creek, CA: AltaMira.

Richardson, R. & Kramer, E. H. (2006). Abduction as the type of inference that characterizes the development of a grounded theory. *Qualitative Research,* 6(4), 497–513.

Schatzki, T. R., Cetina, K. K., & von Savigny, E. (Eds.). (2001). *The practice turn in contemporary theory.* London: Routledge.

Shibutani, T. (1955). Reference groups as perspectives. *American Journal of Sociology,* 60(6), 562–569.

Shibutani, T. (1962). Reference groups and social control. In A. Rose (Ed.), *Human behavior and social processes* (pp. 128–145). Boston: Houghton Mifflin.

Shibutani, T. (1986). *Social processes: An introduction to sociology.* Berkeley: University of California Press.

Shostak, S. (2003). Locating gene-environment interaction: At the intersections of genetics and public health. *Social Science and Medicine*, 56(11), 2327–2342.

Shostak, S. (2005). The emergence of toxicogenomics: A case study of molecularization. *Social Studies of Science*, 35(3), 367–404.

Simon, J. (1996). Discipline and punish: The birth of a middle-range research strategy. *Contemporary Sociology*, 25(3), 316–319.

Star, S. L. (1983). Simplification in scientific work: An example from neuroscience research. *Social Studies of Science*, 13(2), 208–226.

Star, S. L. (1989). *Regions of the mind: Brain research and the quest for scientific certainty.* Stanford, CA: Stanford University Press.

Star, S. L. (1991a). Power, technologies and the phenomenology of conventions: On being allergic to onions. In J. Law (Ed.), *A sociology of monsters: Essays on power, technology and domination* (pp. 26–56). Sociological Review Monograph No. 38. New York: Routledge.

Star, S. L. (1991b). The sociology of the invisible: The primacy of work in the writings of Anselm Strauss. In D. Maines (Ed.), *Social organization and social process: Essays in honor of A. Strauss* (pp. 265–283). Hawthorne, NY: Aldine de Gruyter.

Star, S. L. (1995). The politics of formal representations: Wizards, gurus and organizational complexity. In S. L. Star (Ed.), *Ecologies of knowledge: Work and politics in science and technology* (pp. 88–118). Albany: State University of New York Press.

Star, S. L. (1999). The ethnography of infrastructure. *American Behavioral Scientist*, 43(3), 377–391.

Star, S. L. (2007). Living grounded theory: Cognitive and emotional forms of pragmatism. In A. Bryant & K. Charmaz (Eds.), *Handbook of grounded theory* (pp. 75–94). London: Sage.

Star, S. L. & Strauss, A. L. (1998). Layers of silence, arenas of voice: The ecology of visible and invisible work. *Computer Supported Cooperative Work: The Journal of Collaborative Computing*, 8(1), 9–30.

Strauss, A. L. (1978a). A social worlds perspective. *Studies in Symbolic Interaction*, 1, 119–128.

Strauss, A. L. (1978b). *Negotiations: Varieties, contexts, processes and social order.* San Francisco: Jossey Bass.

Strauss, A. L. (1982a). Interorganizational negotiation. *Urban Life*, 11(3), 350–367.

Strauss, A. L. (1982b). Social worlds and legitimation processes. In N. K. Denzin (Ed.), *Studies in symbolic interaction*, 4th ed. (pp. 171–190). Greenwich, CT: JAI Press.

Strauss, A. L. (1984). Social worlds and their segmentation processes. In N. K. Denzin (Ed.), *Studies in symbolic interaction*, 5th ed. (pp. 123–139). Greenwich, CT: JAI Press.

Strauss, A. L. (1987). *Qualitative analysis for social scientists.* Cambridge: Cambridge University Press.

Strauss, A. L. (1991a). *Creating sociological awareness: Collective images and symbolic representation.* New Brunswick, NJ: Transaction Publishers.

Strauss, A. L. (1991b). Social worlds and spatial processes: An analytic perspective. In W. R. Ellis (Ed.), *A person-environment theory series/The Center for Environmental Design Research Working Paper Series.* Berkeley: Department of Architecture, University of California. Available online at http://sbs. ucsf.edu/medsoc/anselmstrauss/pdf/work-socworlds_spatial.pdf (accessed August 27, 2008).

Strauss, A. L. (1993). *Continual permutation of action.* New York: Aldine de Gruyter.

Strauss, A. L. & Corbin, J. (1990). *The basics of qualitative analysis: Grounded theory procedures and techniques.* Thousand Oaks, CA: Sage.

Strauss, A. L. & Corbin, J. (1994). Grounded theory methodology: An overview. In N. K. Denzin & Y. S. Lincoln (Eds.), *Handbook of qualitative research* (pp. 273–285). Newbury Park, CA: Sage.

Strauss, A. L. & Corbin, J. (Eds.). (1997). *Grounded theory in practice.* Thousand Oaks, CA: Sage.

Strauss, A. L., & Corbin, J. (1998). *The basics of qualitative analysis: Grounded theory procedures and techniques,* 2nd ed. Thousand Oaks, CA: Sage.

Strauss, A. & Fisher, B. (1979). George Herbert Mead and the Chicago tradition of sociology, Part I. *Symbolic Interaction,* 2(1), 9–26.

Strauss, A., Schatzman, L., Bucher, R., Ehrlich, D. and Sabshin, M. (1964). *Psychiatric ideologies and institutions.* Glencoe, IL: The Free Press of Glencoe.

Strübing, J. (2004). *Grounded theory: On the epistemological and social theoretical roots of empirically grounded theory-building.* [*Grounded Theory. Zur sozialtheoretischen und epistemologischen Fundierung des Verfahrens der empirisch begründeten Theoriebildung*] (Series: Qualitative Sozialforschung Vol. 15). Wiesbaden, Germany: VS Verlag für Sozialwissenschaften.

Strübing, J. (2007a). *Anselm Strauss.* Konstanz, Germany: UVK Verlagsgesellschaft mbH.

Strübing, J. (2007b). Research as pragmatic problem-solving: The pragmatist roots of empirically-grounded theorizing. In A. Bryant & K. Charmaz (Eds.), *Handbook of grounded theory* (pp. 580–602). London: Sage.

Thomas, W. I. & Thomas, D. S. [1928] (1970). Situations defined as real are real in their consequences. In G. P. Stone & H. A. Farberman (Eds.), *Social psychology through symbolic interaction* (pp. 154–155). Waltham, MA: Xerox College Publishing.

Wiener, C. L. (1981). *The politics of alcoholism: A social worlds analysis.* New Brunswick, NJ: Transaction Press.

Wiener, C. L. (1991). Arenas and careers: The complex interweaving of personal and organizational destiny. In D. Maines (Ed.), *Social organization and social process: Essays in honor of Anselm Strauss* (pp. 175–188). New York: Aldine De Gruyter.

Wiener, C. L. (2000). *The elusive quest: Accountability in hospitals.* New York: Aldine de Gruyter.

Wiener, C., Strauss, A. Fagerhaugh, S., & Suczek, B. (1992). The AIDS policy arena: Contingent aspects of social world/arena theory. Unpublished ms. Available online at http://sbs.ucsf.edu/medsoc/anselmstrauss/pdf/socworlds-aids.pdf (accessed August 27, 2008).

Woolgar, S. (1991). Configuring the user: The case of usability trials. In J. Law (Ed.), *A sociology of monsters: Essays on power, technology and domination* (pp. 57–102). New York: Routledge.

Dialogue: Questions?

Jan: Adele, Why do you consider your method a type of grounded theory? Your method is so different from the others...

Adele: Well, Jan, I would not say that SA is a type of GT but rather that it is an extension of GT. Specifically, SA assumes that the researcher will do GT coding, memoing and analysis of their data, ideally including analytic diagramming. In addition, researchers will, as appropriate, do theoretical sampling—seek fresh data sources that can "speak" specifically to particular emergent analytic insights, both to deepen them and to provide range of variation. The three kinds of SA maps may be pursued in addition to the GT work.

An interesting question here is at what point in the research process does the analyst ideally do the GT work and the different SA maps. After I finished the SA book, I realized how terrifically the situational maps work as part of the research design stage. They can be done in a flexible way from very initial design through the completion stages of a project. That is, the situational map can and should be constructed *and reconstructed over time* to specify the major elements in the situation of concern about which data need to be gathered, analyzed, and written about.

In terms of using situational maps as part of project design, the key word is emergence. The situational maps are emergent, allowing you to feature and background what you want to, without losing track of potentially important things/issues. The earliest versions are explorer's maps. One of the innovative emphases of SA is that it is not only humans and their organizations that matter today. Many kinds of elements are potentially part of situations. People and things, humans and nonhumans, visual materials, discourses, symbols, controversies, organizations and institutions, each and all can be present *and* mutually consequential.

In contrast, the social worlds/arenas maps and positional maps are usually done further downstream in the research process, especially the positional maps. Both require the analyst to be very familiar with their data and doing some basic GT analytic work is the best way to get there. The social worlds/arenas maps are often a bit easier, or feel that way, because we often have a lot of tacit knowledge about the area we are studying. The positional maps may be more challenging because the analyst has to figure out the axes—not just the topic areas being contested within the discourse but also precisely *how* they are contested—to make the map(s). Their capacity to "help silences speak" by showing what positions are *possible but do not appear in the data* addresses a lack in grounded theory and in many other approaches to qualitative materials.

But these are not hard and fast rules about what should go first or last, more rules of thumb that analysts can violate with aplomb!

8. Grounded Theories
On Solid Ground

Janice M. Morse, Adele E. Clarke, Barbara Bowers, Kathy Charmaz,
Juliet Corbin, and Phyllis Noerager Stern

It is the end of the workshop, and most of the participants have left. Conference staff are moving about the room picking up cups. At the front of the room in the dim lights the workshop participants are discussing the day's sessions. There was general agreement that the day was fun, interesting, and most worthwhile:

Kathy: This was *great*. You know, it is the first time we have sat down together and talked about what we do.

Adele: Yes, but the day was too short—we did not really get a chance to get down to the real similarities and differences in what we actually *do*.

Phyllis: Well this is an opportunity—let's do it now! Jan, get Julie to the phone—no time like the present!

[Julie comes online]

Jan: Hi Julie—We are all here having a postmortem, and thought this would be an opportunity to really discuss where grounded theory is going. Julie—you did not hear all of the sessions today, but do you think we have different grounded theory methods?

Julie: Well, I don't know the exact intricacies of what Kathy and Adele are doing—and they have moved in a different direction, but I think grounded theory is *a way of thinking*. I believe it's a general all-round method, but the way you choose to do it—as long as you have theoretical sampling, constant comparison, ask some sort of questions—*how* you actually do it is individual. We all do it differently. The actual method you use is what works for you. I think you do it differently, Jan. I do it differently, everybody is doing it differently, and that's not important. What is important is that you do "good work."

Phyllis: Well, I use grounded theory strategies as Glaser describes it. I think, you know, if it ain't broke, why fix it? And I haven't read any grounded theory where I have thought "Boy, this is hot stuff!" and they haven't referenced Glaser. The Glaserian method books are available and their number grows annually! I do not believe in recipes for doing research—but these methods are laid out and take the guesswork out of what you are trying to do.

Adele: Yes, but I think there are huge differences in *how* we are doing things differently. The first generation was not feminist, and that is key for me. Both Strauss and Glaser refused to take gender or race or any identity politics into account unless they "earned their way into the analysis." I felt that was an abdication of responsibility for understanding what was going on in the fullest sense possible. People do not talk easily about race, gender and other identity issues. This places a greater burden on the researcher to gather pertinent data. That is not addressed by Glaser or Strauss in the way I am talking about—

Phyllis: You're right! Even though I have adhered to Glaserian grounded theory, I have moved and used feminist and cultural theory in my grounded theory research. If you are doing research in another cultural group—I did a Filipino study—considering the cultural results is an important difference.

Barbara: Of course, we have to be flexible and sensible. But the issue is how much flexibility. Even though Lennie [Schatzman] coauthored his '71 book with Strauss, it was clear to both that he was *not* doing grounded theory. Lennie is an interactionist at heart, and while his position is consistent with symbolic interactionism, his focus is on reasoning and problem-solving in everyday life—you know, basically mapping out all of those things that are a part of the processes, the mundane things that we all engage in during our lives. He is interested in the assumptions and languages used within each discipline or political group. The language gives you the structure of the interaction.

Kathy: Maybe you can call me a "hybrid," because in many ways I have adopted the strategies that Barney Glaser developed, but in a much more Straussian way. I was definitely a student of Strauss, and I have a more open view of what grounded theory can be than Glaser, and have a more open view than even comes across in Strauss and Corbin's (1990, 1998) texts. As we have discussed, emotions (see, for example, Chapter 6 this volume) are really significant in what I do. For me, grounded theory handles social psychological issues very well across the board. But I also think that constructivist grounded theory would be useful for developing social policy/policy analysis, but it has not been used in that area very much. I leave that to the third generation!

Julie: Ah, change! Everything changes—you can't sit around with your head in the sand. Life moves on, new ideas come out. That's the nature of knowledge. You have to respond. But if we really have different kinds of grounded theory—yet sometimes I wonder if we even have such a beast at all—if we do have different kinds of grounded theory, then the differences must be evident in the finished product.

Adele: One problem vis-à-vis situational analysis is that it is so new that we do not have many examples of it in practice yet.

Kathy: Yes, but we have examples in this book of some of these methods. It is interesting for example, to compare the nature of theory developed by Stern in her fire study (Chapter 4, example, this volume), and Bowers and her colleagues (Chapter 5, example, this volume) in the ways they have developed the notion of perspective of care. Both delineate characteristics beautifully; both identify implicit knowledge; both develop theory. But there are differences.

Barbara: I think one of the places we are all moving toward is a greater recognition of the role played by the researcher and the context. I actually had quite an extensive section on that in the manuscript (in *The Gerontologist*), but most of it ended up on the editor's floor. The limitations we face in most journals don't allow much space for reflecting on the context of the research and how that is woven into the study.

Phyllis: In the fire study, the major finding was that there is an absence of grief ritual that is connected to the needs of individuals who have lost their home to fire—the societal response is one of *"No one-was-hurt-and-you-have-insurance-so-I-don't-have-to-do-anything-to-help-you-other-than-tell-you-I'm-sorry."* Whereas Barbara separated out the expectations of nursing home residents, I looked more at context: Under what conditions does this occur, when doesn't it? For example, when people lived in rural areas, they were more likely to be cared for by their neighbors with gifts of food, clothing, and shelter, because rural people depend on one another to survive. Absence of grief ritual is all over the place; think of miscarriage, divorce, burglary. Strangely, burglary is a kind of rape of the security of home.

Adele: That is interesting. And if we take an example from your and Anselm's edited volume of grounded theory studies, Julie—say Orona's (1990) and Kathy's examples (Chapter 6, this volume)—we find important similarities in the descriptive insight and the style of theory presented.

Julie: Yes, Celia Orona's article entitled "Temporality and Identity Loss Due to Alzheimer's Disease" based on her dissertation is an excellent example of a grounded theory study. In her study, she focuses on temporality in the context providing care to persons with Alzheimer's disease. But what is so good about her article is the description she gives of the research process that she went through in developing her grounded theory and her interest in identity loss similar to the work of Charmaz.

Kathy: Constructivist grounded theory builds on earlier forms of the method but also differs from them. To recap some of the points in my Chapter we go deeper into the phenomenon and take it apart starting from the experiencing person's (or persons') perspective rather than that of the analyst. The degree to which a researcher can take an "insider's view" is, of course, relative, but sustained study from as close as the researcher can get to the phenomenon supports gaining an insider's view. In my example, note how I treat surrendering to illness as a significant process to analyze and how my analytic rendering of it conceptualizes the personal accounts.

Phyllis: Now yours is different again Adele. Those situational maps flummox me!

Adele: They can be tricky. To identify everything that's in a situation that you are trying to study, you have to be very broad and deep. Everything in the situation—even the nonhuman—needs to be represented in the map—at least initially. Physical things, people, organizations, buildings, or whatever is in the situation. The project needs to be situated. Some people write up their grounded theory research as though it did not take place in a particular historical time or country or anything—it's sort of abstracted out of itself. I am trying to push things the other way and encourage folks to look at the situation they are interested in much more deeply.

Barbara: You see situation much more differently than context, right?

Adele: A situation is specific—a set of specifications—rather than a general term. What I am actually saying is that there is no such thing as context! Instead, everything that is *inside* the situation broadly conceived is co-constitutive—is part of and produced through everything else—not just "somehow around the edges."

Barbara: I would have made the distinction using the language of condition and context. Condition is the specific aspect of the context that is identified and explored. Context is much larger and remains less specified, but needs to be acknowledged.

Phyllis: Julie said something interesting—she said, we all use theoretical sampling, constant comparison, memo, asking analytic questions of the data. ... Is that correct? Do we all do those things? And what other strategies do we have in common?

Julie: I don't know how you would express the kind of grounded theory thinking—but in the grounded theory I do, its about thinking about process and structure and this has been there since Glaser and Strauss (1967). You see it in their research—take *Awareness of Dying* (Glaser & Strauss, 1965), it's about coming to, and out of, awareness, or maintaining awareness. You can talk about awareness and becoming aware—as a noun or as a gerund. Even if you talk about aware, you have to talk about the strategies and processes, how people become aware, so when we talk about our styles of doing grounded theory, we have to be careful not to split hairs.

I am also worried that how we label our strategies and these may reflect our hair splitting. What is the difference between a core category and a basic social process? Yet Anselm never talked in terms of basic social process. He talks about core category and does not use it in the sense that Barney does.

Barbara: How do you see the differences?

Julie: Well, I've gone back and looked at the books published by Barney and Anselm, for example, *Status Passage* (Glaser & Strauss, 1971), *Patsy and the Subcontractor* (Glaser, 1976), and *Awareness of Dying* (Glaser & Strauss, 1965). Let's take awareness: To me awareness is a core category but not necessarily a process per se. It only takes on the nature of process when Glaser and Strauss start talking about action/interactional strategies used to either maintain a certain level of awareness or move awareness onto the next level. I think the difference is more in terms of semantics than in actual practice because both Glaser and Strauss both look for process and structure and try to locate structure in the larger of context macro conditions. I see the biggest difference, at least it was a difference in the past, but maybe not now, in that Strauss and I don't see data as containing one "theory" only but that it contains the possibility of any different theories. There are a great many researchers from any different disciplines using both Barney's and Strauss's approach to grounded theory in their own ways and doing very high-level and excellent work. People from all over the world are becoming more and more interested in doing grounded theory and using all the books, taking what appeals to them from all approaches to doing grounded theory.

Phyllis: I agree that those are the similarities, and I also agree that a core category is different from the way Barney uses basic social process, but theoretical sampling is theoretical sampling. There is no quarrel there. And constant comparison, developed by Barney, does not come in varieties. The difference there is how far each researcher is willing to push categories to develop the differences in their concepts for phenomena. Barney's math background makes him very fond of 2x2 tables. This probably comes from a different research agenda, but they are useful in Glaserian grounded theory.

Jan: To recap: The differences between each of your styles of grounded theory seem to have come from the different areas of study and the different strategies you have added. Adele's are the most different. Adele, it is my opinion that you have given your approach short shrift! You have something quite unique and very different. But why is it still considered grounded theory?

Adele: Thank you for pushing me, Jan. I see it as both relying on and extending grounded theory. I encourage analysts to code, memo, do analytic diagrams and so on. (The questions at the end of my chapter discuss the possibilities for ordering these.) As for the new strategies I offer, the maps *are* unique. Strauss used social world maps elsewhere—but not linked to grounded theory. He had these as parallel tracks of work, but he did not pull them together. I pulled them together into situational analysis. The situational maps I discussed here are the "big news." The other types of maps—the social worlds/arenas maps and the positional maps—keep the discourses and all the players directly in analytic view. They can be very useful strategies.

But there is another major difference between situational analysis and other grounded theories. I believe you are trying to look for commonalities, right?

Others: Right.

Adele: I try to emphasize the issue of the range of variation and difference. And discourses—visual and historical discourses—as well as understanding documents and whatever preproduced materials that existed before you entered the situation. These materials are very important and have been underutilized by grounded theorists.

Kathy: I think in my view is quite compatible with Dorothy Smith's (1999) notion of "standpoints" and this means recognizing that points of view and ways of doing things come from particular conditions.

Julie: But I think that it all comes down to what grounded theory research looks like at the end. The real test would be to look at the product. How theoretical do you think the end result should be? Or how in depth and well thought out is the analysis. I make a big point of this in the latest *Basics* book (Corbin & Strauss, 2008).

Kathy: That's a good question. I think it depends on the researcher's goals, and not everyone is going for a high conceptual level. Practice and policy people are interested in descriptive studies. I think using grounded theory methods to work on other kinds of problems than theory-building is fine as long as people are clear about their purpose of what they are doing and why they are doing it.

Julie: The early research and Glaser and Strauss monographs were written as elegant monographs in narrative style. Sandelowski (2007) wrote that we go overboard labeling the processes in qualitative research. I think she was referring to grounded theory. If we look at Glaser and Strauss's

Awareness or even Glaser's (1976) *Patsy and the Subcontractor*, we do not see parts of the theory labeled "basic social process" nor do we see it in the title. Now, just because they are not labeled as such, does not mean that social issues are not a part of it. But structure and process are there.

Kathy: Of course, in those monographs—pre-*Discovery* (Glaser & Strauss, 1967)—they may not have had those terms to label those components.

Phyllis: Right! And I think Sandelowski (2007) is wrong. For present-day researchers to remove those labels from their theory would result in both loss of analytic process and organization of the resulting theory. I think those labels are useful!

Adele: Another interesting criticism comes from Paul Atkinson (1997), who argues that the small samples and the in-depth interviewing—without much observational data—places too much emphasis on individuals' experiences and can slant the emerging theory. He thinks we need to attend to what people actually do—not just what they *say* they do.

Kathy: Rich data that speak to the individual's perspective and with impact or meaning (in the phenomenological sense) must come from the interviews. Typically, good interviews are lengthy and consequently data are copious. One cannot have, even with computer-assisted analysis, both in-depth interviews, analyzed interpretively, and a huge sample, analogous to samples for large quantitative surveys! Besides, we cannot always *see* the impact of an ongoing event, for it takes time for these participants to cognitively process whatever is happening and to recognize the impact of the bad news, or whatever.

Jan: A few years ago, Silverman (1998) had some strong criticisms of grounded theorists. He was very critical of their sloppiness in interviews, that is, doing retrospective interviews, rather than fieldwork and recording what people actually said, with all the rigor of conversational analysis notations. I was indignant. How could he be so short sighted? Of course, you have to elicit participant *reports*—that is retrospective data—if you want to get at how people *felt* about something. The emotion that is so important, and can't be always be seen.

Adele: What I thought was odd was that he only addressed grounded theory articles in *Qualitative Health Research* when they are everywhere!

Kathy: His position also misses other important points about grounded theory. The method offers valuable tools for conducting and focusing ethnographic studies and helps ethnographers bring their studies to completion. The lines between ethnography and interviewing blur, too, because ethnographers often rely on conversational interviewing and some draw heavily on formal interviews that they conduct toward the end of their stay in the field setting or afterward. Qualitative researchers who criticize interview methods stress that interviews offer accounts, stories, and reflections, not observed actions. In effect, these critics discount the use of interviews for certain types of research problems. In short, instead of one method being inherently preferable to another, the research problem should direct how researchers collect their data. (Adele cheers loudly.) Part of the debate on interviewing rests on a realist's quest for truth, rather than on establishing a range of theoretical possibilities, consistent with grounded theory practice.

To engage criticisms of grounded theory, we need to look at what its critics address. These critics often conflate the *method* itself with how various researchers have used it, or claim to have used it. Antony Bryant (2002) has termed the latter, the "grounded theory mantra"; it serves as a form of legitimation of method, not use or explication of it. And some researchers view grounded theory as an expedient tool for accruing publications. Unfortunately, numerous studies that researchers have done in the name of grounded theory offer little analysis, rely on limited empirical data, and ignore relevant literatures. Yet grounded theory studies shine when researchers gather extensive rich data, offer original ideas about these data, establish solid evidence for their ideas, and recognize the range and limits of these ideas.

Phyllis: We know that grounded theory is not easy—it is very difficult—and poor grounded theory is simply obvious rubbish. The major problems I see as an editor are inadequate data (from too small sampling and lack of theoretical sampling, lack of saturation, and a lack of a comparison of data), resulting in obvious findings. Good grounded theory surprises and delights—this is the "grab" that Glaser was talking about. Sometimes I send submitted manuscripts back to the authors, saying "You are not finished yet—collect more data!" or "More comparison will give your work life." Sometimes the problem is dissertations written in article format, and too many articles coming from one study.

Julie: Oh, everyone wants a doctorate! And you have got to do research and write a publishable paper, but not necessarily to put the hard effort into the work. ... So. ...

Barbara: But what grounded theory application? It is not enough to tell others what our participants are thinking. Why isn't grounded theory more useful? We seldom see application and even rarer still evaluation.

Phyllis: I think they are unsure what to do with it.

Jan: Some time ago, I developed a method of converting grounded theory results to an assessment guide (Morse, Hutchinson & Penrod, 1998). It works very well, and the next step from this is intervention and evaluation. But it has not happened for some reason. ...

Barbara: We work with a different kind of evidence and a different kind of knowledge. ... Maybe the world is not ready yet.

Jan: Speaking of the world not being ready, where is grounded theory going?

Adele: I think one direction that is really important is paying attention to the non-human things in social life and attending to how they affect the situations we study. Take medical technologies for example. How do people engage technologies like the birth control pill or a Pap smear? Monica Casper (1998) looked at how different professional groups fought over and divided the turf related to fetal surgery. What does the Internet mean for how we understand our illnesses and diseases? It is not just people out there, and global warming brings home this point all too vividly.

Barbara: You are right Adele. But what are you are doing is a life's work! It's very important, and has profound implications. But you need a research team and collaborators with common research interests, yet in different disciplines. There is certainly room for this research.

I am interested in working on methods, perhaps looking at the influence of the researcher-as-an-instrument. And we need to figure out how to develop a mentoring program for other researchers. I am working with some folks in Australia—it seems to be going well.

Julie: We have gone a full circle. This one thing the Anselm did well—he was a mentor par excellence! We are still learning from him!

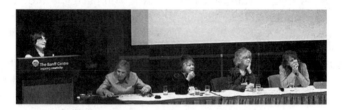

The Banff Symposium panel, seated left to right: Phyllis Noerager Stern, Adele E. Clarke, Kathy Charmaz and Barbara Bowers. Janice M. Morse, Podium. Juliet Corbin was on the phone. Photo by Mary Barros-Bailey, PhD, Boise, Idaho.

References

Atkinson, P. (1997). Narrative turn or a blind alley? *Qualitative Health Research*, 7(3), 325–344.

Bryant, A. (2002). Re-grounding grounded theory. *The Journal of Information Technology Theory and Application*, 4, 25–42.

Casper, M. (1998). *The making of the unborn patient : a social anatomy of fetal surgery*. New Brunswick, NJ: Rutgers University Press.

Charmaz, K. (2006). *Constructing grounded theory*. London: Sage.

Clarke, A. (2005) *Situational analysis: Grounded theory after the postmodern turn*. Thousand Oaks, CA: Sage.

Corbin, J. & Strauss, A. L. (2008). *Basics of qualitative research*. Thousand Oaks, CA: Sage.

Glaser, B. G. (1976). *Experts versus laymen: A study of the patsy and the subcontractor*. Mill Valley, CA: Sociology Press.

Glaser, B. G. & Strauss, A. L. (1965). *Awareness of dying*. Chicago: Aldine.

Glaser B. G. & Strauss, A. L. (1967). *Discovery of grounded theory*. Chicago: Aldine.

Glaser, B. G., & Strauss, A. L. & (1971). *Status passage: A formal theory*. Chicago: Aldine.

Morse, J. M., Hutchinson, S., & Penrod, J. (1998). From theory to practice: The development of assessment guides from qualitatively derived theory. *Qualitative Health Research*, 8, 329–340.

Orona, C. (1990). Temporality and identity loss due to Alzheimer's disease. *Social Science & Medicine*, 10, 1247–1256. Reprinted in A. L. Strauss & J. Corbin (Eds.) (1997). *Grounded theory in practice* (pp. 171–196). Thousand Oaks, CA: Sage.

Sandelowski, M. (2007). Words that should be seen, but not written. *Research in Nursing and in Health* [Editorial], 30, 129–130.

Schatzman, L. & Strauss, A. L. (1971). Field research. Englewood Cliffs, NJ: Prentice-Hall.

Silverman, D. (1998). The contested character of qualitative research. In D. Silverman (Ed.), *Doing qualitative research: A practical handbook* (pp. 283–297). London: Sage.

Smith, D. E. (1999). *Writing the social: Critique, theory, and investigations.* Toronto: University of Toronto Press.

Strauss, A. L. & Corbin, J. (1990). *Basics of qualitative research: Grounded theory procedures and techniques.* Newbury Park, CA: Sage.

Strauss, A. L. & Corbin, J. (1998). *Basics of qualitative research: Techniques and procedures for developing grounded theory*, 2nd ed. Newbury Park, CA: Sage.

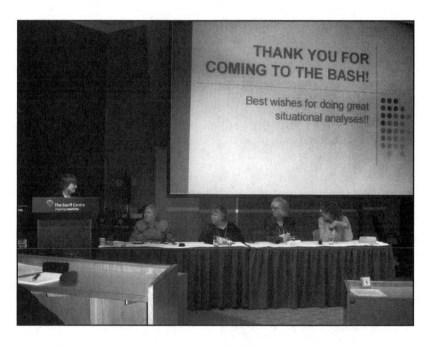

Left to right: Janice M. Morse, Phyllis Noerager Stern,
Adele E. Clarke, Kathy Charmaz, and Barbara Bowers

Resources

In this section, we list the publications of Glaser and Strauss that have not been previously cited in this volume, other resources (some fast becoming classics in their own right), grounded theory methods books, and key articles written for specific disciplines, monographs that use grounded theory, and foreign-language titles and translations.

Grounded Theory Methods

Glaser and/or Strauss

Corbin, J. (1991). Anselm Strauss: An intellectual biography. In D. Maines (Ed.), *Social organization and social process: Essays in honor of Anselm Strauss* (pp. 17–42). Hawthorne, NY: Aldine de Gruyter.

Corbin, J. & Strauss, A. L. (1990). Grounded theory research: Procedures, canons, and evaluative criteria. *Qualitative Sociology*, 13(1), 3–21.

Corbin, J., & Strauss, A. L. (1996). Analytic ordering for theoretical purposes. *Qualitative Inquiry*, 2(2), 139–150.

Corbin, J. & Strauss, A. L. (2008). *Basics of qualitative research*, 3rd ed. Thousand Oaks, CA: Sage.

Glaser, B. G. (1978). *Theoretical sensitivity.* Mill Valley, CA: Sociology Press.

Glaser, B. G. (1992). *Emergence versus forcing: Basics of grounded theory analysis.* Mill Valley, CA: Sociology Press.

Glaser, B. G. (1993). *Examples of grounded theory: A reader.* Mill Valley, CA: Sociology Press.

Glaser, B. G. (1994). *More grounded theory methodology: A reader.* Mill Valley, CA: Sociology Press.

Glaser, B. G. (1995). *Grounded theory: 1984–1994.* Mill Valley, CA: Sociology Press.

Glaser, B. G. (with the assistance of W. D. Kaplan) (1996). *Gerund grounded theory: The basic social process dissertation.* Mill Valley, CA: Sociology Press.

Glaser, B. G. (1998). *Doing grounded theory: Issues and discussions.* Mill Valley, CA: Sociology Press.

Glaser, B. G. (2001). *The grounded theory perspective: Conceptualization contrasted with description.* Mill Valley, CA: Sociology Press.

Glaser, B. G. (2003). *The grounded theory perspective II: Description's remodeling of grounded theory.* Mill Valley, CA: Sociology Press.

Glaser, B. G. (2005). *The grounded theory perspective III: Theoretical coding.* Mill Valley, CA: Sociology Press.

Glaser, B. G. (2006). *Doing formal grounded theory: A proposal.* Mill Valley, CA: Sociology Press.

Glaser, B. G. & Holton, J. A. (Eds.). (2007). *The grounded theory seminar reader.* Mill Valley, CA: Sociology Press.

Glaser, B. G. & Strauss, A. L. (1967, 1999). *The discovery of grounded theory: Strategies for qualitative research.* Chicago: Aldine.

Strauss, A. L. (1987). *Qualitative analysis for social scientists.* Cambridge, UK: Cambridge University Press.

Strauss, A. L. (1995). Notes on the nature and development of general theories. *Qualitative Inquiry,* 1(1), 7–18.

Strauss, A. L. & Corbin, J. (1990). *Basics of qualitative research.* Thousand Oaks, CA: Sage.

Strauss, A. L. & Corbin, J. (1991). Tracing lines of conditional influence: Matrix and paths (1990). In A. L. Strauss (Ed.), *Creating sociological awareness: Collective images and symbolic representation* (pp. 455–464). New Brunswick, NJ: Transaction Publications.

Strauss, A. L. & Corbin, J. (1994). Grounded theory methodology: An overview. In N. K. Denzin and Y. S. Lincoln (Eds.), *Handbook of qualitative research* (pp. 273–285). Newbury Park, CA: Sage.

Strauss, A. L. & Corbin, J. (Eds.). (1997). *Grounded theory in practice.* Thousand Oaks, CA: Sage.

Strauss, A. L. & Corbin, J. (1998). *Basics of qualitative research,* 2nd ed. Thousand Oaks, CA: Sage.

Glaser and Strauss Research Monographs

Crabtree, D. J. & Glaser, B. G. (1961). *Second deeds of trust: How to make money safely.* Mill Valley, CA: Sociology Press.

Glaser, B. G. (1968). *Organizational careers: A sourcebook for theory.* Chicago: Aldine.

Glaser, B. G. (1976). *Experts versus laymen: A study of the patsy and the subcontractor.* Mill Valley, CA: Sociology Press.

Glaser, B. G. & Strauss, A. L. (1965). *Awareness of dying.* Chicago: Aldine.

Glaser, B. G. & Strauss, A. L. (1970). *Anguish: Case study of a dying patient.* San Francisco: Sociology Press.

Glaser, B. G. & Strauss, A. L. (1974). *Time for dying.* Chicago: Aldine.

Glaser, B. G. & Strauss, A. L. (1975). *Chronic illness and the quality of life.* Chicago: Aldine.

Strauss, A. L. (1959). *Mirrors and masks: The search for identity.* Glencoe, IL: Free Press. [1997 New edition with a new Introduction by Anselm L. Strauss. New Brunswick, NJ: Transaction Publishers.]

Strauss, A. L. (1978). *Negotiations: Varieties, contexts, processes, and social order.* San Francisco: Jossey-Bass.

Strauss, A. L., Fagerhaugh, S., Suczek, B. & Wiener, C. (1985). *The social organization of medical work.* Chicago: University of Chicago Press. [1997 New edition with a new introduction by Anselm L. Strauss. New Brunswick, NJ: Transaction Publishers.]

Strauss, A. L., Schatzman, L. Bucher, R. Ehrlich, D. & Sabshin, M. (1964). *Psychiatric ideologies and institutions.* Glencoe, IL: The Free Press. [1981 New edition with a new Introduction. New Brunswick, NJ: Transaction Publishers.]

Grounded Theory Methods: Other Authors (not in this volume)

Bryant, T. & Charmaz, K. (2007). *Handbook of grounded theory.* London: Sage.

Chenitz, W. C. & Swanson, J. (1986). *From practice to grounded theory.* Menlo Park, CA: Addison Wesley.

Dahlgren, L., Emmelin, M., & Anna Winkvist. (2007). *Qualitative methodology for international public health.* Umea, Sweden: International School of Public Health, Umea University.

Dey, I. (1999). *Grounding grounded theory: Guidelines for qualitative inquiry.* San Diego, CA: Academic Press.

Locke, K. (1996). Rewriting the discovery of grounded theory after 25 years? *Journal of Management Inquiry,* 5(1), 239–245.

Locke, K. (2001). *Grounded theory in management research.* Thousand Oaks, CA: Sage.

Konecki, K. (2000). *Studies in Qualitative Methodology: Grounded Theory* (in Polish). Warsaw, Poland: PWN.

Koniecke, K. (Ed.). (2002). *Qualitative Sociological Review.* Available online at http://www.qualitativesociologyreview.org/ENG/index_eng.php (accessed September 9, 2008).

Maines, D. (Ed.). (1991). *Social organization and social process: Essays in honor of Anselm Strauss.* Hawthorne, NY: Aldine de Gruyter.

O'Connor, M. K., Netting, F. E. Netting, & Thomas, M. L. (2008). Grounded theory: Managing the challenge for those facing institutional review board oversight. *Qualitative Inquiry*, 14(1), 28–45.

Schreiber, R. S. & Stern, P. N. (Eds.). (2001). *Using grounded theory in nursing.* New York: Springer.

Wilson, H. S., & Hutchinson, S. A. (1996). Methodologic mistakes in grounded theory. *Nursing Research*, 45, 122–124.

Selected Grounded Theory Research Monographs and Collections

Ekins, R. (1997). *Male femaling: A grounded theory approach to cross-dressing and sex-changing.* Foreword by A. L. Strauss. London: Routledge.

Kearney, M. (1999). *Understanding women's recovery from illness and trauma.* Thousand Oaks, CA: Sage.

Melia, K. M. (1987). *Learning and working: The occupational socialization of nurses.* London: Tavistock.

Morse, J. M., & Johnson, J. L. (Eds.). (1991). *The illness experience: Dimensions of suffering.* Newbury Park, CA: Sage. Available online at http://content.lib.utah. edu/u?/ir-main,2008 (accessed June 15, 2008).

May, K. (Ed.). (1996). Advances in grounded theory (Special Issue). *Qualitative Health Research*, 6(3), 309–441.

Foreign Language Titles and Translations

Charmaz, K. (2006). *Constructing grounded theory.* London: Sage. Chinese translation: Chongqing University Press, Chonqing. Japanese translation by Hisako Kakai and Kiyoko Sueda, Kyoto, Japan: Nakanishiya Shuppan. Portuguese translation: Artmed Editora, Port Alegre, Brazil, 2007.

Clarke, A. E. (2005) *Situational analysis: Grounded theory after the postmodern turn.* Thousand Oaks, CA: Sage. Simplified Chinese translation: Chongqing University Press, Chonqing.Glaser, B. G. & Strauss, A. L. (1965). *Awareness of dying.* Chicago: Aldine. London: Weidenfeld and Nicolson, 1973. The Netherlands, German translation: *Interaktion mit Sterbenden: Beobachtungen für Ärzte, Schwestern, Seelsorger und Angehörige.* Göttingen, Germany: Vandenhoeck & Ruprecht (Sammlung Vandenhoeck), 1974.

Glaser, B. G. & Strauss, A. L. (1967). *The discovery of grounded theory.* Chicago: Aldine. London: Weidenfeld and Nicholson. German translation: Alphen aan de Tijn: Samson, 1976. Japanese translation by Setsuo Mizuno, 1996.

Koniecke, K. (2000). *Studies in qualitative methodology: Grounded theory* [in Polish]. Warsaw, Poland: PWN.

Schatzman, L. & Strauss, A. L. 1973. *Field research: Strategies for a natural sociology*. Englewood Cliffs, NJ: Prentice-Hall. Japanese translation by Takao Kawai. Tuttle-Mori"Agency, Tokyo, 1999.

Schreiber, R. S. & Stern, P. N. (2001). *Using grounded theory in nursing*. New York: Springer. Korean translation: Hyunmoonsa Publishers, 2003.

Strauss, A. L. (1984). *Feldtheorie-Grundzüge der Grounded Theory*. Hagen, Germany: University of Hagen.

Strauss, A. L. (1987). *Qualitative analysis for social scientists*. New York: Cambridge University Press. (1991). *Grundlagen qualitativer sozialforschung: Datenanalyse und theoriebildung in der empirischen soziologischen forschung*. Translated by Astrid Hildenbrand; Foreword by Bruno Hildenbrand. Munich, Germany: Wilhelm Fink Verlag. German.

Strauss, A. L. (1992). *La trame de la negociation: Sociologie qualitative et interactionnisme* [The web of negotiation: Qualitative sociology and interactionism]. Edited by I. Baszanger with her introduction of Strauss's work and his own introduction to the French translation. Paris: L'Harmattan. For the English translation of Strauss's introduction, see his website at http://sbs.ucsf.edu/medsoc/anselmstrauss/ (accessed August 28, 2008).

Strauss, A. L. (2004). *Grounded theory*. Zur sozialtheoretischen und epistemologischen Fundierung des Verfahrens der empirisch begründeten Theoriebildung Grounded Theory: [On the epistemological and social theoretical roots of empirically grounded theory-building]. Series: Qualitative Sozialforschung, vol. 15. Wiesbaden, Germany: VS Verlag für Sozialwissenschaften.

Strauss, A. L. & Corbin, J. (1990). *Basics of qualitative research: Grounded theory procedures and techniques*. Newbury Park, CA: Sage. Korean translation: Hanual Publishing, 1995. German translation: Weimheim: Beltz, Psychologie Verlags Union, 1996. Chinese translation: Chu Liu Book Company, 1997. Arabic translation: Kingdom of Saudi Arabia, Institute of Public Administration, 1999. Japanese translation: Igaku-Shoin Ltd., Tokyo, 1999. Russian translation, YPCC, Mockba, 2001.

Strauss, A. L. & Corbin, J. (1994). *Basics of qualitative research*. Psychologie Verlags Union, Germany. Kingdom of Saudi Arabia, Institute of Public Administration, Arabic, 1995. Chu Liu Book Company Chinese, Chinese, 1995. Hanual Publishing, Korean, 1995. Sdruzeni Podane Ruce, Czech, 1998. Editions Universitaires, French, 1998. Editorial URSS, Russian, 2001. Igaku-Shoin, Ltd., Japanese, 1995 and 2003. Artmed Editora Portuguese, Portugal, 2004.

Strauss, A. L. & Corbin, J. (1998). *Basics of qualitative research*, 2nd ed. Thousand Oaks, CA: Sage. Czech translation: Sdruzeni Podane Ruce, 1998. French translation: Editions Universitaires, 1998. Chinese translation: Waterstone Pubs., 2001. Russian translation, Editorial URSS, 2001. Spanish translation, Colombia: Facultad de Enfermeria de la Universidad de Antioquia, Editorial Universidad de Antioquia, 2002. Japanese translation: Igaku-Shoin, Ltd., 2003. Portuguese translation: Artmed Editora, 2004.

Strübing, J. (2004). *Grounded theory. Zur sozialtheoretischen und epistemologischen fundierung des verfahrens der empirisch begründeten theoriebildung* [Grounded theory: On the epistemological and social theoretical roots of empirically grounded theory-building]. Series: Qualitative Sozialforschung, vol. 15. Wiesbaden, Germany: VS Verlag für Sozialwissenschaften.

Strübing, J. (2007). *Anselm Strauss.* Konstanz, Germany: UVK Verlagsgesellschaft mbH.

Index

Abductive reasoning, 137
Abstract situational maps
    messy, 212
    ordered, 213
Actants (in SA), 203–205
    implicated, 204
    nonhuman, 203
Actions, 156
    in constructivist GT, 131
    and intentions, 158
    research, 38
Activity levels, 156
Adapting
    to impairment, 157–158
    to loss, 157
Adler, N., 33
Albrecht, G., 156, 173, 186
Allen, M., 60
Aller, L. J., 107, 108, 122
Analytic process, 43–50, 57
    and perspective, 97
Analysis
    everyday, 101
    stage, 161
    subjectivity in, 192–193
Anguish: Case Study of a Dying Patient
    (1970), 26
Applbaum, K., 203, 224
Arenas (SA), 199
Ashworth, P. D., 107, 122
Atkinson, P., 135, 138, 150, 214, 224, 243
Attitudes, 156
Awareness of Dying (1965), 25
Axial coding, 138

Baker, C., 68, 81
Basic Social Process, 9, 240
Basics of Qualitative Research (1st ed., 1990),
    36, 37, 38, 53, 154

Basics of Qualitative Research (2nd ed., 1998),
    36, 37, 53
Basics of Qualitative Research (3rd ed., 2008),
    36, 41, 51, 53
Baszanger, I., 223, 224
Becker, H. S., 223, 224
Beisser, A. R., 161, 180, 186
Bennett, L. A. (see Wolin)
Benoliel, J. Q., 25, 29, 60, 64
Bijker, W., 202, 224
Bliesmer, M., 107, 122
Blumer, H., 23, 29, 39, 40, 53, 150, 186, 197,
    202, 224
Bowers, B. (also see Schatzmar), 11, 17, 18,
    20–21, 24, 54, 85, 86–106, 107–124, 122,
    125, 126, 192, 193, 236–246
    bibliography, 263–265
    biography, 263
Bowker, G., 150
Boychuk Duchscher, J. E., 150
Bright, M. A., 71, 81
Brocklehurst, J., 108, 122
Brody, H., 155, 186
Brooke, V. M., 108, 122
Brown, M. A., 87, 104
Bruce, J., 204, 224
Bryant, A., 128, 135, 136, 149, 150, 222, 224,
    244, 246
Bucher, R., 223, 224
Burawoy, M., 150
Burke, P., 158, 186
Bury, M., 155, 186

Care, 107–124
    as comfort, 117–119
    patient-centered, 107
    as relating, 115–117
    as service, 113–115
Caron, C., 18, 87, 104, 122

Carson, P. P., 108, 122
Casper, M. J., 130, 132, 140, 142, 146, 150, 223, 224, 245
Categories, 44
Chafer, S., 26
Charmaz, K., 11, 16, 17, 18, 21, 24, 25, 37, 53, 54, 56, 63, 64, 84–85, 127–154, 155–191, 192, 197, 198, 222, 225, 236–246
  bibliography, 266–268
  biography, 265
  in photo album, 31, 34Chicago School of Sociology, 9, 88, 198–199, 205
Cisneros-Puebla, C. A., 135, 151
Clark, P., 108, 122
Clarke, A., 16, 17, 19, 21, 24, 25, 37, 53, 64, 130, 135, 140, 148, 150, 192, 194–233, 236–246
  bibliography, 270–271
  biography, 195–196, 269
  in photo album, 31, 34
Classical GT, 137
  as objectivist GT, 140–141
Cleary, P. D., 108, 122
Clifford, J., 152
Coding, 40–41
  axial, 138
  in emergence, 138
  in the "fire study," 70
  as a thinking process, 41
Coeling, H. V. (see Aller)
Coffey, A. (see Atkinson)
Comforting ritual
  absence of, 61
Comparative analysis, 90, 91
  in Straussion GT, 95
  valuing dimensions, 92
Concepts, 61
  basis for discourse, 40
  basis for understanding, 40
  building, 48
  disciplinary, 99
  foundation of GT, 52
  inverted, 38
  properties of, 44
Conceptualizing, 39
Conditional matrix, 60, 208–210
  Clarke's 2005, 209
  Strauss & Corbin's (1990), 207
  Strauss & Corbin's (1998), 208
Conjuring, 93
Context, 238–239
  cf situation, 240
Cooley, C. H., 158, 187Constant comparison, 61, 68
Constructionist, 39, 63, 129ff
Constructivist GT
  action in, 131
  assumption, 130
  comparison with objectivist GT, 140–146
  definition, 129–130

epistemological ground, 129
  meaning, 131, 132, 144
  ontological ground, 131–132
  social construction in, 130
  steps in, 162
Covan, E. K., 23, 55, 63, 64
Corbin, J., 15, 16, 17, 19, 24, 25, 28, 29, 35–53, 54, 135, 162, 165, 187, 206, 223, 232, 236–249
  bibliography, 271–274
  biography, 271
  evolving GT, 35
  masters thesis, 36
  in photo album, 32
Core variable/category, 63, 68, 241
  cf basic social process, 240
Creative
  process, 57
  researcher, 43

Dangdomyouth, P., 57, 64
Data, 56
  accuracy, 58
  cleaning, 54
  as constructed vs. discovered, 131
  discovery of, 138
  dynamic nature of, 42
  guided by questions, 45
  statistical, 57
  trust of, 59
Dahlberg, C. C., 173, 187
Dahlgren, L., 226
Davies, A. R., 108, 122
Davis, F., 24
Davis, M. A., 122
Davis, S.
  photo album, 30
Davis-Floyd, R., 71, 90
Dawson, L., 162, 187
DeBeauvoir, S., 194, 227
Deconstruction
  criticism of, 206
Deegan, M. J., 204, 227
Delmont, S. (see Atkinson)
Denzin, N. K., 37, 53, 158, 162, 178, 181, 200, 225
Derugin, L., 31
Devore, D. J., 87, 105
Dewey, J., 221, 227
Dey, I., 56, 64, 214, 227
Dickenson, E. (see Brocklehurst)
DiGiacomo, S. M., 187
Dimensional algorithm, 126
Dimension analysis, 85–106, 108–124
  assumptions, 103
  conjuring, 93
  convergence with GT, 90
  definition, 95
  disciplinary concepts, 100
  emergence of, 16

learning, 99–101
natural analysis, 102
perspective, 97–98
purpose of, 90
study of nursing students, 96
Dimensions
assigning relative value, 94
in complexity of social life, 95
Dimensions of experience, 93
Dingwall, R., 187, 199, 227
Discourses, 142
in SA, 200
Discovery of Grounded Theory (1967), 9, 11, 15, 25, 41, 53, 56, 62, 64, 68, 89, 105, 122, 128, 148, 205, 228
Doka, K. J., 144, 152
Donabedian, A., 108, 122
Donnally, T., 170, 187
Dreyfus, H. L., 201, 227
DuBois, W. E. B., 204, 227
Dugdale, A., 201
Dunning, J., 221, 227
Durkheim, E., 152

Earle, P. (see Bliesmer)
Emergence, 36, 59, 138
emerging perspective, 100
Emotions, 54, 243
in interviewing, 193
in research, 38
Ericsson, S., 152
Ethnography, 13
comparison with GT, 9
to examine experience, 108
Experience
analysis in, 101
dimensions of, 93
giving meaning, 39
of nursing home, 110
response to, 39
Esmond, S. (see Bowers), 87, 106

Fabrega, H., 160, 187
Fallowfield, L., 187
Festchrift, 16
Fibich, B., 107
Field notes, 58
Fine, G. A., 199, 227
Fisher, G. C., 161, 164, 187
Fit, 61
Flood, M. E., 24, 26, 29
Ford, P. (see Welsh)
Formal theory, 62
Fosket, J. R., 220, 227Foucault, M., 200, 201, 202, 227
Fourth International Congress on Women's Health Issues, 56
Frank, A. W., 158, 161, 165, 167, 179, 187, 188
Frankenberg, R., 158, 188
Freund, P., 158, 188
Friedson, G., 223, 228

Friese, C., 220, 228Fujimura, J., 134, 152, 223, 228

Gadow, S., 155, 158, 163, 188
Garrety, K., 223, 228
Gerhardt, U., 188
Gerteis, M., 107, 123
Gilles, C. L. (see Kools)
Glaser, B. G., 15, 19, 29, 59, 64, 79, 89, 129, 148, 152, 160, 195, 228, 237
biography, 24–25
as a mentor, 62
photo album, 30
Glaser & Strauss, 9, 23, 24, 194
characteristics of classic GT, 137
contrasting positions, 128
developers of GT, 15, 17, 18
Discovery, 9, 11, 15, 68
interpersonal styles, 26, 28
interpretation of, 55
interpreting data, 59
students of, 9, 16
working with students, 22
Glaserian Grounded Theory, 15–16, 17, 55–65, 237
Glasner, B., 158, 164, 188
Goffman, E., 108, 123, 159, 188
Grab, 61
Grant, N. K., 107, 123
Grau, L., 107, 108, 123
Grief, 144–145
disenfranchised grief, 144
entitled grief, 145
Grounded theory (GT)
compendium of methods, 41
computers, 17
data, 56
development of the idea, 56
diligence in, 129
doing, 20–22
epistemological ground, 129–133
epistemological underpinnings, 139
evolved, 63
as a "general method," 127–128
method, 42
objectivist GT, 137, 142
ontological ground, 129–133
positivistic, 58
process of, 20, 60
purpose of, 13–14
questioning as a method, 41
questions about emergence, 17
sampling in, 20
shifting views of, 133
statistics, 57
types of, 16–77
"way of thinking about data," 14
"Grounded Theory Bash" Banff Symposium, 9, 194
Gubrium, J., 108, 123

Hall, P., 200, 207, 228
Hamberg, K., 40, 53
Hamilton, R., 87, 105
Haraway, D., 136, 143, 152, 203, 223, 228
Health Care for Women International, 61
Hearn, J., 203, 228
Henwood, K. 128, 152,
Herzlich, C., 156, 163, 188
Hewitt, J. P., 158, 188
Hildenbrand, B., 206, 228
Hodder, I., 228
Holton, J. A., 28, 56
Home loss by fire, 66–83
Hoschchild, A., 149
Huey, F. L., 71, 81
Hughes, G. C., 40, 53, 199, 228
Hutchinson, S., 74, 81
Huttmann, B., 71, 85
Hypotheses, 68

Identity
    changing goals, 173–176
Image (see *Journal of Nursing Scholarship*)
Impairment
    adapting to, 157–158
Inferring
    about dimensions, 94
Interactionist perspective, 38
Internet, 46
Interpretation, 39
    in constructivist GT, 131
    in data analysis, 63
    legitimate, 40
    trying out, 43
Interviews
    about Vietnam War, 46–48
    ethics of, 84–85

Jackson, J. L., 108, 123
Jackson, M. M., 71, 81
Jacobson, N. (see Bowers), 107
Jenks, C., 197, 228
Jirovec, M. M., 107, 123
Joffe, C., 215, 219, 228
Johansson, E. (see Hamberg)
Johnson, C. L., 188
Journal of Nursing Scholarship, 55, 56

Kacperczyk, A., 220, 229
Kahane, D. H., 162, 188
Kane, R. A., 107, 123
Karp, D., 132–133, 153, 185, 188, 189
Keane, A., 79, 80, 81
Kearney, M. H., 135, 153, 229
Kelle, U., 135, 149, 153
Kelly, M., 162, 188
Kerry, J. (see Stern), 70, 81
Kestenbaum, V., 159, 189
Kezar, A., 148, 153
Kidel, M., 179, 189
Knowledge

in constructivist GT, 130
    development, 39
    knowledge-based practice, 40
Kools, S., 87, 105
Kotorba, J., 158, 189
Kubler-Ross, E., 161, 189
Kurtz, L. R., 199

Laitinen, P., 108, 123
Larsson, B. W., 108, 123
Lather, P., 196, 229
Latour, B., 202, 229
Law, J., 202, 223, 229
Layder, D., 135, 153
Lazersfeld, P., 24
Lehr, H., 123
LeMaistre, J., 161, 179, 189
Lengnick-Hall, C. A., 108, 123
Liang, H., 87, 105
Lilrank, A., 54
Lindemann, E., 70, 78, 81
Lindesmith, A., 188
Literature
    use of, 62, 63
Locke, K., 135, 153, 214, 229
Locker, D., 159, 189
Lofland, J., 161, 189
Longmate, M. A. (see Ashworth)
Ludwig-Beymer, P., 108, 123
Lutz, B. J., 87, 105, 107, 123

MacDonald, L., 159, 189
Mairs, N., 161, 189
Manning, P. K., 184, 189
Mapping situations, 239
    abstract, 211
    positional maps, 210
    situational maps, 210
    social world/arenas, 210
Marcus, G. (see Clifford), 153, 229
Mattiasson, A-C., 107, 124
Maxwell, E. K. (see Coven), 55, 65, 71, 80, 82
Maxwell, R. J. (see Maxwell, E. K.)
May, K., 135, 149, 153
McCarthy, D., 202, 229
McCarthy, M. C., 87, 105, 106
Mead, G. H., 23–24, 29, 128, 153, 158, 189, 229
Meaning, 38
    and experience, 39
    in constructivist GT, 131, 144
Melia, K. M., 148, 153
Meltzer, B. N., 198, 229
Memoing, 60, 84, 126
Menton, R. K., 24
Messy situational map, 212
Method
    GT method, 51–52
    questioning GT as a method, 41
Miller, D., 203, 229

Miller, N. A., 124
Mills, C. W., 210, 220, 230
Mills, J., 153
Mitchell, P., 108, 124
Monks, J., 155, 167, 179, 189
Morse, J. M., 13–19, 61, 72, 82, 236–249
    bibliography, 275–276
    biography, 274
Murphy, R., 155, 161, 164, 176, 189
Murphy, S. A., 78, 79, 82

Nader, L., 148, 153
Namh, H., 24
National Citizens Coalition for Nursing
    Home Reform, 107, 124
National Fire Investigation, 67
Natural analysis, 102
Nelkin, D., 200, 230
Nores, T. H., 107, 124
Norton, S., 87, 106
Northrup, D. T., 67, 70, 76, 82
Nursing Students, study of
    using dimensional analysis, 96

Objective
    research as, 37
Objectivist GT, 137–142
    and abstraction, 138
Objectivity, 57
O'Connor, M. K., 222, 230
Odendahl, T., 148, 153
Olesen, V., 24, 26, 40, 53, 158, 162, 184, 190,
    196, 230
Olier, M. D., 71, 82
Olshansky, E. F. (see Brown), 87, 106
Online Archives of California Anslem
    Strauss, 29
Ordered situational map, 212
Orona, C., 239, 247
Ostrander, S., 148, 153
Oudshoorn, N., 205, 230
Owens, D. J., 108, 124

Pandhi, N., 63, 65
Park, R. E., 40, 53, 199, 202, 230
Participants' responses
    action, 38
    to emotions,
    to experience, 39
    to meaning, 39
    to research, 38
Patient-centered care, 107
Pearson, A., 107, 108, 124
Peirce, C. S., 137, 138, 153
Perceptions
    as equality indicator, 108
Perspective
    in analysis, 99
    for assessing quality, 108
    in constructivist, 131
    in dimensional analysis, 97-98

emergent, 100
Peters, D. A., 124
Peyrot, M. J. F., 190
Pfeffer, E., 106
Phenomenology
    influence of GT, 60
Pitzele, S. K., 161, 173, 190
Plough, A. L., 190
Positional maps, 210
Practice
    knowledge-based, 40
Pragmatist perspective, 38, 128
Prior, L., 201, 230
Process, 60
Prosono, M.
    photo album, 33
Prus, R. C., 162, 190
Publishing
    prematurely, 84
Purser, M., 184

Qualitative Analysis for Social Scientists
    (Strauss, 1984), 15, 89, 125, 154, 232
Qualitative research
    background, 36
Qualitative synthesis, 62
Quality assurance, 107
Quality of care
    characteristic, 109
Quint, J. (see Benoliel)

Radley, A., 156, 158, 175, 179, 190
Reality
    in findings, 37
    multiple, 38
Recognition recall, 125
Reflexive analysis, 40, 129, 133
Register, C., 161, 164, 190
Reichert, J., 137, 153, 214, 230
Research
    actions, 38
    context, 38
    interactionist perspective, 38
    pragmatist perspective, 38
Research methods
    altering and adapting, 17
    copyright?, 18
    standardized vs. changing, 18
Research question
    relationship to data collection, 134
Researcher
    being creative, 43
    contemporary ideas about, 38
    creating distance, 125
    formulating questions, 51
    "going native," 37
    objective, 37
Researcher distance, 125
Resources
    foreign language, 254–256
    GT methods, 251–252

GT research, 254
Glaser & Strauss monographs, 252
other authors, 253–254
Reynolds, L., 197, 230
Richardson, R., 214, 230
"Ritual support connections," 66, 71–75
Robinson, I., 185, 190
Rosenkoetter, M. M., 63, 65
Rosenthal, G., 137, 154

Sampling (see also Theoretical Sampling), 69
Sandelowski, M., 242, 267
Sanders, C. R., 158, 190
Sanders, S., 58
Schatzki, T. R., 203, 230
Schatzman, L., 16, 18, 19, 24, 85–106, 124, 125, 196, 237, 247
biography, 87–90
photo album, 30, 31, 32, 33, 34
Scheela, R. A., 82
Schmah, J., 71, 82
Schwandt, T. A., 38, 39, 53
Seidman, I. E., 161, 190
Shibutani, T., 230
Shilling, C., 159, 190
Shostak, S., 220, 231
Silverman, D., 243, 247
Simon, J., 200, 231
Situational Analysis (SA), 16, 194–232
actants, 204–205
arenas, 199
conceiving, 196–233
conditional matrix, 205–210
discourse in, 200
nonhuman object, 201
situational maps, 210–212, 234–235
as a theory/methods package, 191
Situational maps, 210, 234
abstract, 212
examples, 215–219
messy, 212
ordered, 212
relational, 219
Social context, 173–176
Social psychological processes, 68
Social structural processes, 68
Social Worlds/Arena's maps, 210
Sociology Press, 16, 27, 28, 59, 60
Speedling, E., 190
Stage analysis, 161
Star, S. L. (see Bowker), 134, 154, 195, 197, 199, 223
Statistics in GT, 56
Status Passage (1971), 26, 62
Stepfather study, 57
Stephens, N., 148, 154
Stern, P. N., 11, 15, 17, 19, 27, 28, 55–65, 192, 236–246
bibliography, 276–279
biography, 27, 276

Sternian Grounded Theory, 56
Strauss, A. L., 15, 16, 17, 19, 23–25, 43, 82, 124, 152, 154, 160, 162, 165, 190, 191, 195, 196, 197, 206, 222, 223, 228, 231
association with Schatzman
biography, 23–24
photo album, 30, 31, 32
Straussian Grounded Theory, 15–16, 17, 42, 238
Strong, M., 184, 191
Strubing, J., 214, 232
"Studying up," 148
Subjectivity, 192–193
Substantive theory, 62
Symbolic interactionism, 61, 134
perspective on identity, 158

Techniques
as a tool, 40
Thai caregivers, 57
Thematic analysis, 20–21
Theoretic sampling, 48, 49
Theoretical code, 61
Theoretical sensitivity, 125
Theoretical Sensitivity (Glaser, 1978), 15, 27, 148, 152
Theory
formal, 62
relationship to data, 36
substantive theory, 62
Theory-driven analysis, 88
Thomas, W. I., 40, 53, 210, 232
Time dimensions, 75
stage analysis, 161
Time for Dying (1968), 26
Transcribing, 192–193
Transcripts, 54
Truth, 37
Turner, B., 159, 191

UCSF (University of California of San Francisco), 10, 13, 16, 21, 23, 25, 55, 196
mentors in, 36
School of Nursing, 59, 88

Vietnam War, 42–50

Walin, S., 71, 83
Walker, D., 154
Walker, V., 71, 82, 83
Watson, K. C., 87, 106
Weitz, R., 164, 191
Wetle, T., 108, 124
Wiener, C. L., 222, 232
Williams, R. G. A., 156, 163, 191
Wilson, H., 56, 59, 65
Wolf, Z., 71, 83
Woolgar, S., 202, 233
Wuest, Judy, 61, 63, 65

Yoshida, K. K., 162, 191

Zola, I. K., 158, 191

About the Authors

Barbara Bowers

Dr. Bowers is the associate dean for Research and Sponsored Programs, the Helen Denne Schulte Professor, and the director, Center for Excellence in Long-Term Care, University of Wisconsin–Madison School of Nursing. She also has an adjunct position at the Australian Catholic University, Melbourne. She obtained her BS in nursing from the University of Michigan, Ann Arbor, an MS from Wayne State University, Detroit, and the PhD in sociology from the University of California, San Francisco (UCSF).

Her association with Lenny Schatzman began during her tenure as a predoctoral student at UCSF. She was the first of Lenny's students to use dimensional analysis as the research method for her dissertation. Spending many hours in Lenny's office—as his thoughts about dimensional analysis evolved and staying in close contact with Lenny over the subsequent years—has given her a close-up view of the methodology and how it can be used. Although Schatzman continues to work on his book about dimensional analysis, the methodology has remained largely within the oral realm, precluding productive discussion and debate about it.

Bibliography

Bowers, B. J. (1987). Intergenerational caregiving: Adult caregivers and their aging parents. *Advances in Nursing Science*, 9(2), 20–31.

Bowers, B. J. (1988). Family perceptions of care in nursing homes. *The Gerontologist*, 28(3), 361–368.

Bowers, B. (1989). Grounded theory: From conceptualization to research process. In B. Sarter (Ed.), *Paths to knowledge: Innovative research methods in nursing* (pp. 33–58). New York: National League of Nursing.

Bowers, B. J. (1996). *The relationship between staffing and quality in long-term care facilities*. Report to the 105th U.S. Congress, Subcommittee on Health: Appropriateness of Minimum Nurse Staffing Ratios.

Bowers, B. J. (2005). Foreword. In J. Gaugler (Ed.), *Promoting family involvement in long-term care settings* (pp. xi–xiii). Baltimore: Health Professions Press.

Bowers, B. J. & Becker M. (1992). Nurse aides in nursing homes: The relationship between organization and quality. *The Gerontologist*, 32(3), 360–366.

Bowers, B. J., Esmond, S. L., & Canales, M. (1999). Approaches to case management supervision. *Administration in Social Work*, 23(1), 29–49.

Bowers, B. J., Esmond, S. L., & Jacobson, N. (2000). The relationship between staffing and quality in long-term care facilities: Exploring the views of nurse aides. *Journal of Nursing Care Quality*, 14(4), 55–64.

Bowers, B. J., Esmond, S. L., & Jacobson, N. (2003). Turnover reinterpreted: CNAs talk about why they leave. *Journal of Gerontological Nursing*, 29(3), 36–43.

Bowers, B.J., Esmond, S. L., Norton, S., & Holloway, E. (2006). The consumer/provider relationship as care quality mediator. In S. Kunkel & V. Wellin (Eds.), *Consumer voice and choice in long-term care* (ch. 10). New York: Springer.

Bowers, B. J., Fibich, B., & Jacobson, N. (2001). Care as service, care as relating, care as comfort: Understanding nursing home residents' perceptions of quality. *The Gerontologist*, 41(4), 539–545.

Bowers, B. J., Lauring, C., & Jacobson, N. (2001). How nurses manage time and work in long-term care facilities. *Journal of Advanced Nursing*, 33(4), 484–91.

Caron, C. & Bowers, B. J. (2000). Methods and application of dimensional analysis: A contribution to concept and knowledge development in nursing. In B. L. Rodgers & K. A. Knafl (Eds.), *Concept development in nursing, foundations, techniques and applications* (pp. 285–319). Philadelphia: W.B. Saunders.

Caron, C. D. & Bowers, B. J. (2003). Deciding whether to continue, share or relinquish caregiving: Caregiver views. *Qualitative Health Research*, 13(9), 1252–1271.

DeVore, D. J. & Bowers, B. J. (2006). Childcare for children with disabilities: Families search for specialized care and cooperative childcare partnerships. *Infants & Young Children*, 19(3), 203–212.

Hamilton, R. & Bowers, B. J. (2005). Disclosing genetic test results to family members. *Journal of Nursing Scholarship*, 37(1), 18–24.

Hamilton, R. & Bowers, B. J. (In press). Convergence of age, genetic risk, and treatment decisions in young women (18–39y/o) at risk for hereditary breast and ovarian cancer. *Genetics in Medicine*.

Lutz, B. & Bowers, B. J. (2000). Patient-centered care: Understanding its interpretation and implementation in health care. *Journal of Scholarly Inquiry for Nursing Practice*, 14(2), 183–187.

Lutz, B. & Bowers, B. J. (2005). The influence of disability on everyday life. *Qualitative Health Research*, 15(8), 1037–1054.

Lutz, B., Bowers, B. J., Esmond, S. L., & Jacobson, N. (2003). Improving primary care for persons with disabilities: The nature of expertise. *Disability & Society*, 18(4), 443–455.

Norton, S. & Bowers, B. J. (2001). Working toward consensus: Providers' strategies to shift patients from curative to palliative treatment choices. *Research in Nursing & Health*, 24(4), 258–269.

Pandhi, N., Bowers, B. J., & Chen, F. (2007). A comfortable relationship: A patient derived dimension of ongoing care. *Family Medicine*, 39(4), 266–273.

Tluczek, A., Mischler, E., Bowers, B. J., Peterson, N., Morris, M., Farrell, P., Bruns, N., Colby, H., McCarthy, C., Fost, N., and Carey, P. (1991). Psychological impact of false-positive results when screening for cystic fibrosis. *Pediatric Pulmonology*, 7, 29–37.

Kathy Charmaz

Kathy Charmaz earned her BS in occupational therapy from the University of Kansas, Lawrence, her MA in sociology from San Francisco State College, and a PhD in sociology from UCSF in 1973. Since 1981, she has been professor of sociology at Sonoma State University, California, where she teaches courses in classical sociological theory, medical sociology, and social psychology. She also heads the Faculty Writing Program in which she works with faculty on their research and writing.

Dr. Charmaz has written extensively about grounded theory and served as the editor of *Symbolic Interaction* from 1999 to 2003. As developer of "constructivist grounded theory," she has integrated the classic grounded theory guidelines of Barney Glaser and Anselm Strauss with methodological developments of the past forty years. Constructivist grounded theory is a fundamentally interactive and comparative method that adopts a relativist view of the research situation and the researcher's standpoints as well as of empirical realities. Dr. Charmaz's version of grounded theory takes the method further into interpretive social science.

Bibliography

Bryant, A. & Charmaz, K. (2007). Grounded theory in historical perspective: An epistemological account. In A. Bryant & K. Charmaz (Eds.), *Handbook of grounded theory* (pp. 31–57). London: Sage.

Bryant, A & Charmaz, K. (Eds.). (2007). *Handbook of grounded theory.* London: Sage.

Bryant, A. & Charmaz, K. (2007). Introduction. In A. Bryant and K. Charmaz (Eds.), *Handbook of grounded theory* (pp. 1–28). London: Sage.

Calkins, K. (1970). Time: Perspectives, marking and styles of usage. *Social Problems,* 17(4), 487–501.

Calkins, K. (1972). Shouldering a burden. *Omega,* 3(1), 16–32. Reprinted in 1976, R. A. Kalish (Ed.), *Caring relationships* (pp. 73–86). Farmingdale, NY: Baywood.

Charmaz, K. (1975). The coroner's strategies for announcing death. *Urban Life,* 4(3), 296–316. Reprinted in 1977, L. H. Lofland (Ed.), *Toward a sociology of death* (pp. 296–316). Beverly Hills, CA, Sage.

Charmaz, K. (1980). The social construction of self-pity in the chronically ill. In N. K. Denzin (Ed.), *Studies in symbolic interaction,* vol. 3 (pp. 123–145). Greenwich, CT: JAI Press.

Charmaz, K. (1983). Loss of self: A fundamental form of suffering in the chronically ill. *Sociology of Health and Illness,* 5(2), 168–195.

Charmaz, K. (1983). The grounded theory method: An explanation and interpretation. In R. M. Emerson (Ed.), *Contemporary field research* (pp. 109–126). Boston: Little Brown.

Charmaz, K. (1987). Struggling for a self: Identity levels of the chronically ill. In P. Conrad & J. Roth (Eds.), *Research in the sociology of health care, the experience of chronic illness,* vol. 6 (pp. 283–232). Greenwich, CT: JAI Press.

Charmaz, K. (1989). The self in time. In N. K. Denzin (Ed.), *Studies in symbolic interaction,* vol. 10 (pp. 127–141). Greenwich, CT: JAI Press.

Charmaz, K. (1990). "Discovering" chronic illness: Using grounded theory. *Social Science and Medicine,* 30(11), 1161–1172.

Charmaz, K. (1991). *Good days, bad days: The self in chronic illness and time.* New Brunswick, NJ: Rutgers University Press.

Charmaz, K. (1991). Turning points and fictional identities. In D. R. Maines (Ed.), *Social organization and social processes: Essays in honor of Anselm Strauss* (pp. 71–86). New York: Aldine.

Charmaz, K. (1994). "Discoveries" of self in illness. In M. L. Dietz, R. Prus, & W. Shaffir (Eds.), *Doing everyday life: Ethnography as lived experience* (pp. 226–242). Mississauga, Ontario: Copp Clark Longman.

Charmaz, K. (1994). Identity dilemmas of chronically ill men. *Sociological Quarterly,* 35(2), 269–288.

Charmaz, K. (1995). Between positivism and postmodernism: Implications for methods. In N. K. Denzin (Ed.). *Studies in symbolic interaction*, vol. 17 (pp. 43–72). Greenwich, CT: JAI Press.

Charmaz, K. (1995). Grounded theory. In J. A. Smith, R. Harre, & L. Van Langenhove (Eds.), *Rethinking methods in psychology* (pp. 27–49). London: Sage.

Charmaz, K. (1995). The body, identity and self: Adapting to impairment. *The Sociological Quarterly*, 36(4), 657–680.

Charmaz, K. (1996). Time and identity: The shaping of selves of the chronically ill. In B. G. Glaser with W. D. Kaplan (Eds.), *Gerund grounded theory: The basic social process dissertation* (pp. 29–41). Mill Valley, CA: Sociology Press.

Charmaz, K. (1999). Keynote address: Stories of suffering: Subjects' tales and research narratives. *Qualitative Health Research*, 9(9), 369–382.

Charmaz, K. (2000). Grounded theory methodology: Objectivist and constructivist qualitative methods. In N. K. Denzin & Y. S. Lincoln (Eds.), *Handbook of qualitative research*, 2nd ed. (pp. 509–535). Thousand Oaks, CA: Sage.

Charmaz, K. (2000). Presidential address: Looking backward, moving forward: Expanding sociological horizons in the twenty-first century. *Sociological Perspectives*, 43(4), 527–549.

Charmaz, K. (2000). Teachings of Anselm Strauss: Remembrances and reflections. *Sociological Perspectives* (Supplemental Issue), 43, S163–S174.

Charmaz, K. (2002). Grounded theory: Methodology and theory construction. In N. J. Smelser & P. B. Baltes (Eds.), *International encyclopedia of the social and behavioral sciences* (pp. 6396–6399). Amsterdam: Pergamon.

Charmaz, K. (2002). Grounded theory analysis. In J. F. Gubrium & J. A. Holstein (Eds.), *Handbook of interview research* (pp. 675–694). Thousand Oaks, CA: Sage. Reprinted in J. A. Holstein & J. F. Gubrium (Eds.), *Inside interviewing: New lenses, new concerns*. Thousand Oaks, CA: Sage.

Charmaz, K. (2002). Stories and silences: Disclosures and self in chronic illness. *Qualitative Inquiry*, 8(8), 302–328.

Charmaz, K. (2002). The self as habit: The reconstruction of self in chronic illness. *The Occupational Therapy Journal of Research*, 22 (Supplement 1), 31s–42s.

Charmaz, K. (2003). Grounded theory. In M. Lewis-Beck. A. E. Bryman & T. F. Liao (Eds.), *The Sage encyclopedia of social science research methods* (pp. 440–444). London: Sage.

Charmaz, K. (2003). Grounded theory. In J. A. Smith (Ed.), *Qualitative psychology: A practical guide to research methods* (pp. 81–110). London: Sage.

Charmaz, K. (2004). Keynote address: Premises, principles, and practices in qualitative research: Revisiting the Foundations. *Qualitative Health Research*, 14(7), 976–993.

Charmaz, K. (2005). Grounded theory in the 21st century: Applications for advancing social justice studies. In N. K. Denzin & Y. S. Lincoln (Eds.), *Handbook of qualitative research*, 3rd ed. (pp. 507–535). Thousand Oaks, CA: Sage.

Charmaz, K. (2006). *Constructing grounded theory: A practical guide through qualitative analysis.* London: Sage.

Charmaz, K.(2006). Grounded theory. In G. Ritzer (Ed.), *Encyclopedia of sociology IV* (pp. 2023–2027). Cambridge, MA: Blackwell.

Charmaz, K. (2006). Measuring pursuits, marking self: Meaning construction in chronic illness. *International Journal of Qualitative Health and Well-Being,* 1(1), 27–37.

Charmaz, K. (2007). Constructionism and grounded theory. In J. A. Holstein and J. F. Gubrium (Eds.), *Handbook of constructionist research* (pp. 319–412). New York: Guilford.

Charmaz, K. (2007). Tensions in qualitative research. *Sociologisk Forskning,* 2(1), 76–85.

Charmaz, K. (2008). Grounded theory. In J. A. Smith (Ed.), *Qualitative psychology: A practical guide to research methods,* 2nd ed. (pp. 81–110). London: Sage. (Revised and updated version of the 2003 chapter.)

Charmaz, K. (2008). Grounded theory as an emergent method. In S. Hesse-Biber and P. Leavy (Eds.), *The handbook of emergent methods* (pp. 155–170). New York: Guilford.

Charmaz, K. (2008). Keynote address. Views from the margins: Voices, silences, and suffering. *Qualitative Psychology,* 5(1), 7–18.

Charmaz, K. (2008). The Legacy of Anselm Strauss in Constructivist Grounded Theory. In N. K. Denzin (Ed.), *Studies in symbolic interaction,* 32, 125–139. Bingley, UK: Emerald Publishing Group, Ltd.

Charmaz, K. (2008). Reconstructing grounded theory. In P. Alasuutari, L. Bickman, & J. Brannen (Eds.), *Handbook of social research methods* (pp. 461–478). London, Sage.

Charmaz, K. (Forthcoming). Recollecting Good and Bad Days. In W. Shaffir, A. Puddephatt, & S. Kleinknecht (Eds.), *Ethnographies revisited: The stories behind the story.* New York: Routledge.

Charmaz, K. (Forthcoming). Stories, silences, and self: Dilemmas in disclosing chronic illness (expanded version). In D. Brashers & D. Goldstein (Eds.), *Health communication.* New York: Lawrence Erlbaum.

Charmaz, K. & Bryant, A. (Forthcoming). Grounded theory. In L. M. Given (Ed.), *The Sage encyclopedia of qualitative research methods.* Thousand Oaks, CA: Sage.

Charmaz, K. & Henwood, K. (2008). Grounded theory in psychology. In C. Willig & W. Stainton-Rogers (Eds.) *Handbook of qualitative research in psychology* (pp. 240–259). London: Sage.

Charmaz, K. & Mitchell, R. G. (2001). Grounded theory in ethnography. In P. Atkinson, A. Coffey, S. Delamont, J. Lofland, & L. H. Lofland (Eds.), *Handbook of ethnography* (pp. 160–174). London: Sage.

Adele E. Clarke

Adele E. Clarke did her undergraduate work at Barnard College, New York, a Master's in sociology at New York University, her PhD at UCSF with Anselm Strauss, and a postdoc in organizations at Stanford with Richard Scott. She is currently professor of sociology and history of health sciences at UCSF. She has taught the qualitative research methods sequence of courses there since 1990 and has published works on qualitative research in German, French, and English. Her book *Situational Analysis: Grounded Theory after the Postmodern Turn* (Sage, 2005) offers an extension of the grounded theory method focused on mapping strategies. It won the 2006 Charles Horton Cooley Award of the Society for the Study of Symbolic Interaction. Dr. Clarke's research has centered on studies of science, technology, and medicine, with special emphasis on common medical technologies for women such as the Pap smear, contraception, and RU486. Her major work has been on the formation of the American reproductive sciences in biology, medicine, and agriculture, including *Disciplining Reproduction: American Life Scientists and the "Problem of Sex"* (University of California Press, 1998), which won the Eileen Basker Memorial Prize given by the Society for Medical Anthropology, and the Ludwig Fleck Award of the Society for Social Studies of Science. She also coedited a volume focused on scientific practice titled *The Right Tools for the Job: At Work in Twentieth Century Life Sciences* (Princeton University Press, 1992; French translation by Synthelabo Press: Paris, 1996). In women's health, Clarke has coedited *Women's Health: Complexities and Diversities* (Ohio State University Press, 1997) and *Revisioning Women, Health and Healing: Cultural, Feminist and Technoscience Perspectives* (Routledge, 1999).

Clarke's recent work has focused on biomedicalization—the expansion of biomedicine into increasing areas of life (human and nonhuman) through implementing diverse technoscientific innovations. With a team of colleagues, she has published on this in the *American Sociological Review* (2003) and edited *Biomedicalization: Technoscience and Transformations of Health and Illness in the U.S.*, a volume of case studies. Her next projects center on reproductive technologies, women's health movements, and global health.

Bibliography

Clarke, A. E. (1991). Social worlds theory as organizational theory. In D. Maines (Ed.), *Social organization and social process: Essays in honor of Anselm Strauss* (pp. 119–158). Hawthorn, NY: Aldine de Gruyter.

Clarke, A. E. (2002). Neue wege der qualitativen forschung und die grounded theory [New directions in qualitative methods and grounded theory]. In D. Schaegger (Ed.), *Qualitative gesundheits und pflegeforschung [New directions in qualitative health research]* (pp. 71–89). Bern, Switzerland: Verlag Hans Huber.

Clarke, A. E. (2003). Situational analyses: Grounded theory mapping after the postmodern turn. *Symbolic Interaction*, 26(4), 553–576.

Clarke, A. E. (2005). *Situational analysis: Grounded theory after the postmodern turn.* Thousand Oaks, CA: Sage.

Clarke, A. E. (2006). Feminisms, grounded theory and situational analysis. In S. Hesse-Biber (Ed.), *The handbook of feminist research: Theory and praxis* (pp. 345–370). Thousand Oaks, CA: Sage.

Clarke, A. E. (2006). Social worlds. In G. Ritzer (Ed.), *The Blackwell encyclopedia of sociology* (pp. 4547–4549). Malden MA: Blackwell.

Clarke, A. E. (2007). Grounded theory: Conflicts, debates and situational analysis. In W. Outhwaite & S. P. Turner (Eds.), *Handbook of social science* (pp. 838–885). Thousand Oaks, CA: Sage.

Clarke, A. E. (2008). Sex/Gender and Race/Ethnicity in the Legacy of Anselm Strauss. In Special Section: Celebrating Anselm Strauss and Forty Years of Grounded Theory, in N. K. Denzin (Ed.), *Studies in Symbolic Interaction*, 32, 159–174.

Clarke, A. E. (In press). Anselm L. Strauss. In G. Ritzer (Ed.), *The Blackwell encyclopedia of sociology.* Malden, MA: Blackwell.

Clarke, A. E. (In press). On *Getting Lost* with Patti Lather. *Frontiers: A Journal of Women's Studies.* Available online atjournal is located at Arizona State U. & published by Johns Hopkinds but neither is usually included in a citation. Website is http://www.asu.edu/clas/asuhistory/frontiers/?q=frontiers/' (accessed September 15, 2008)

.Clarke, A. E. (In press, in French). Sex/Gender and Race/Ethnicity in the Legacy of Anselm Strauss: Gender and work in the scholarship of Anselm Strauss. In D. Chabaud-Rychter, V. Descoutures, A. Devreux, & E. Varikas (Eds.), *Genre, travail, mobilités: Questions de genre aux sciences sociales "normâles"* [The gender question in mainstream sociology]. Paris: La Découverte.

Clarke, A. E. (In press). Situational analysis: A Haraway-inspired feminist approach to qualitative research. In S. Ghamari-Tabrizi (Ed.), *Thinking with Donna Haraway.* Cambridge, MA: MIT Press.

Clarke, A. E. & Montini, T. (1993). The many faces of RU486: Tales of situated knowledges and technological contestations. *Science, Technology and Human Values*, 18(1), 42–78.

Clarke, A. E. & Friese, C. (2007). Situational analysis: Going beyond traditional grounded theory. In K. Charmaz & A. Bryant (Eds.), *The handbook of grounded theory* (pp. 694–743). London: Sage.

Clarke, A. E. & Star, S. L. (2007). Social worlds/arenas as a theory-methods package. In E. J. Hackett, O. Amsterdamska, M. Lynch, & J. Wajcman (Eds.), *The handbook of science and technology studies*, 3rd ed. (pp. 113–137). Cambridge, MA: MIT Press.

Juliet Corbin

Julie Corbin collaborated with Anselm Strauss for sixteen years. She received her BSN from Arizona State University, Tempe, her MSN from San Jose State University, a DNSc from UCSF, and served as a postdoctoral research fellow in the Department of Social and Behavioral Sciences, UCSF. She holds a position as senior scientist at the IIQM, University of Alberta, Canada, and is a visiting professor at Salford University, Manchester, England. She retired from formal teaching in 1999 but continues to work with students on an individual basis, offer workshops on grounded theory method, and give selected presentations.

Dr. Corbin was also a family nurse practitioner and held a position as lecturer at San Jose University. She has presented keynote addresses and workshops on grounded theory methods internationally. She has received numerous awards for her research, including Nurse Scholar of the Year Award from Thomas Jefferson University and from Sigma Theta Tau, and the Book of the Year Award from the *American Journal of Nursing.*

Bibliography

Corbin, J. (1982). Protective governing: Strategies for managing a pregnancy combined with a chronic illness. Doctoral dissertation, San Franscico: UCSF.

Corbin, J. (1986). Coding, writing memos, and diagramming. In C. Chenitz & J. Swanson (Eds.), *Qualitative research in nursing* (pp. 102–120). Menlo Park, CA: Addison-Wesley.

Corbin, J. (1986). Qualitative analysis for grounded theory. In C. Chenitz & J. Swanson (Eds.), *Qualitative research in nursing* (pp. 91–101). Menlo Park, CA: Addison-Wesley.

Corbin, J. (1987). Women's perceptions and management of a pregnancy compli- cated by chronic illness. *Health Care for Women International*, 8, 317–337.

Corbin, J. (1990). Balancing resource demand against supply: Maintaining qual- ity of life in the elderly chronically ill. In C. Chenitz, J. Takano-Stone, & S. A. Salisbury (Eds.), *The clinical practice of gerontological nursing* (pp. 547–555). Philadelphia: J.B. Saunders.

Corbin, J. (1991). Anselm Strauss: An intellectual biography. In D. Maines (Ed.), *Social organizations and social process* (pp. 17–42). Hawthorn, NY: Aldine.

Corbin, J. (1992). The caregiving trajectory: An interactive processual frame- work. *Revue Internationale D'action Communautaire* (International Review of Community Development), 28/68, 39–49.

Corbin, J. (1994). Response to the article operationalizing the Corbin and Strauss trajectory model. *Scholarly Inquiry for Nursing Practice*, 7(4), 265–268.

Corbin, J. (1996). Rehabilitation: A biographical medical process. In T. Schott, B. Badura, H-J. Schwager, P. Wolf, & P. Wolters (Eds.), *Neue Wege in der Reha- bilitation* (pp. 174–181). Weinheim, Germany: Juventa Verlag.

Corbin, J. (1998). The Corbin and Strauss chronic illness trajectory model: An update. *Scholarly Inquiry for Nursing Practice: An International Journal*, 12(1), 33–41.

Corbin, J. (1999). Kritische Analyse von Ergebnissen der Plegeforschung. Werkvertrag für Studienbrief (Modul). Jena, Germany: FH Jena Fachbereich Sozialwesen.

Corbin, J. (1999). Response to "Analysis and evaluation of the trajectory theory of chronic illness management." *Scholarly Inquiry for Nursing Practice*, 13(2), 105–109.

Corbin, J. & Hildenbrand, B. (2000). Qualitative Forschung. In B. Rennen-Allhoff & D. Schaeffer (Eds.), *Handbuch Pflegewissenschaft* (pp. 159–186). Weinheim, Germany: Juventa.

Corbin, J. & Morse, J. M. (2003). The unstructured interactive interview: Issues of reciprocity and risks. *Qualitative Inquiry*, 9 (3), 335–354.

Corbin, J. & Strauss, A. L. (1984). Collaboration: Couples working together to manage chronic illness. *Image*, 6(4), 109–115.

Corbin, J. & Strauss, A. L. (1985). Managing chronic illness at home: Three lines of work. *Qualitative Sociology*, 8(3), 224–247.

Corbin, J. & Strauss, A. L. (1985). Issues concerning regimen management in the home. *Ageing and Society*, 5, 249–265.

Corbin, J. Strauss, A. (1987). Accompaniments of chronic illness changes in body, self, biography and biographical time. *Research in the Sociology of Health Care*, 6, 249–281.

Corbin, J. & Strauss, A. L. (1988). Ted and Alice. *Nursing Times*, 84(14), 32–33.

Corbin, J. & Strauss, A. L. (1988). *Unending work and care: Management of chronic illness at home.* San Francisco, CA: Jossey Bass. German translation, R. Piper GmbH & Co. 1993.

Corbin, J. & Strauss, A. L. (1988). Working together. *Nursing Times*, 84(13), 48–49.

Corbin, J. & Strauss, A. L. (1990). Grounded theory research: Procedures, cannons, and evaluative criteria. *Qualitative Sociology*, 13(1), 3–21. Reprinted in *Zeitschrift für Soziologie ZfS*. 19(6), 418–427.

Corbin, J. & Strauss, A. L. (1990). Making Arrangements: The key to home care. In J. F. Gubrium & A. Sankar (Eds.), *The home care experience, ethnography and policy* (pp. 59–73). Newbury Park, CA: Sage.

Corbin, J. & Strauss, A. L. (1991). A nursing model for chronic illness management based upon the trajectory framework. *Scholarly Inquiry for Nursing Practice*, 4(3), 155–174.

Corbin, J. & Strauss, A. L. (1991). Comeback: Overcoming disability. In G. Albretch & J. Levy (Eds.), *Advances in medical sociology*, vol. 2 (pp. 137–159). Greenwich, CT.: JAI Press.

Corbin, J. & Strauss, A. L. (1992). A nursing model for chronic illness management based upon the trajectory framework. In P. Woog (Ed.), *The chronic illness trajectory framework: The Corbin and Strauss nursing model* (pp. 9–28). New York: Springer.

Corbin, J. & Strauss, A. L. (1993). Work and interaction. *The Sociological Quarterly*, 34(1), 71–83.

Corbin, J. & Strauss, A. L. (1994). A chronic illness management framework based upon the trajectory framework. In Japanese translation of P. Woog (Ed.), *The chronic illness trajectory framework: The Corbin and Strauss nursing model*. Tokyo: Igaku-Shoin.

Corbin, J. & Strauss, A. L. (1996). Analytic ordering for theoretical purposes. *Qualitative Inquiry*, 2(2), 139–140.

Strauss, A. L. & Corbin, J. (1988). *Shaping a new health care system*. San Francisco, CA: Jossey Bass.

Strauss, A. L. & Corbin, J. (1990). *Basics of qualitative research*. Newbury Park, CA: Sage. Chinese translation, Taiwan: Chu Liu Book Co, 1997. Japanese translation, Tokyo: Igaku-Shoin Ltd., 1999. Saudi Arabian translation, Riyadh: Kingdom of Saudi Arabia, Institute of Public Administration, 1999.

Strauss, A. L. & Corbin, J. (1994). Grounded theory methodology: An overview. In N. K. Denzin & Y. S. Lincoln (Eds.), *Handbook of qualitative research* (pp. 273–285). Newbury Park, CA: Sage.

Strauss, A. L. & Corbin, J. (1995). *Grounded theory: Grundlagen Qualitativer Sozialforschung*. German translation, translated by H. Legewie. Weinheim, Germany: Beltz, Psychologie Verlags Union.

Strauss, A. L. & Corbin, J. (Eds.) (1997). *Grounded theory in practice.* Newbury Park, CA: Sage.

Strauss, A. L. & Corbin, J. (1998). *Basics of qualitative research*, 2nd ed. Thousand Oaks, CA: Sage.

Strauss, A., Corbin, J., Fagerhaugh, S., Glaser, B. G., Maines, D., Suczek, B., & Wiener, C. (1984, 2ⁿᵈ ed.). *Chronic illness and the quality of life*. St. Louis: C.V. Mosby. Japanese translation, Nursing Book Publishing Department, Igaku-Shoin Ltd., Tokyo, Japan, 1984.

Janice M. Morse

Janice Morse, as organizer of the Grounded Theory Bash, is the only member of the session who has not been a protégée of either Barney Glaser or Anselm Strauss; nor did she attend UCSF. She has, however, conducted grounded theory since the mid-1980s and has observed the developments in grounded theory with interest.

Janice Morse received her BS and MS (nursing) from Pennsylvania State University, University Park, and her MA and PhD (anthropology) and PhD (nursing) from the University of Utah, Salt Lake City. She is presently a professor and Barnes Presidential Chair at the University of Utah, and Professor Emerita, University of Alberta. She was at the University of Alberta for twenty years, where she established and served as the founding director and scientific director of the International Institute for Qualitative Methodology and founding editor of the *International Journal of Qualitative Methods*. She also served as professor at Pennsylvania State University. She is founding editor of *Qualitative Health Research* (Sage Publications), now in Volume 19.

In 1991, Morse and Joy Johnson published *The Illness Experience: Dimensions of Suffering*, a collection of six grounded theories, and the last chapter in this book—"The Illness Constellation Model"—became one of the first meta-analyses in qualitative inquiry. Since then, Morse has used grounded theory with a number of topics, including breastfeeding, and various studies exploring the illness experience.

Bibliography

Estabrooks, C. & Morse, J. M. (1992). Toward a theory of touch: The touching process and acquiring a touching style. *Journal of Advanced Nursing*, 17, 448–456. Reprinted in J. P. Smith (Ed.), 1994, *Models, theories, and concepts* (pp.

ABOUT THE AUTHORS

71–87), London: Blackwell Science Publishers, and in B. Glaser (Ed.), (1995), *Grounded theory 1984–1994*, vol 1. (pp. 301–316), Mill Valley, CA: Sociology Press.

Hupcey, J. E., Penrod, J., & Morse, J. M. (2000). Establishing and maintaining trust during acute care hospitalizations. *Scholarly Inquiry for Nursing Practice: An International Journal*, 14(3), 227–242.

Johnson, J. L. & Morse, J. M. (1990). Regaining control: The process of adjustment following myocardial infarction. *Heart and Lung*, 19(2), 126–135.

Morse, J. M. (1989). Gift-giving in the patient-nurse relationship: Reciprocity for care? *Canadian Journal of Nursing Research*, 21(1), 33–46.

Morse, J. M. (1991). Negotiating commitment and involvement in the patient-nurse relationship. *Journal of Advanced Nursing*, 16, 455–468. Reprinted in 1992, in J. M. Morse (Ed.), *Qualitative health research* (pp. 333–360). Menlo Park, CA: Sage.

Morse, J. M. (1997). Fragmenting theory: On publishing parts of the whole [Editorial]. *Qualitative Health Research*, 8(1), 5–6.

Morse, J. M. (1997). Responding to threats to integrity of self. *Advances in Nursing Science*, 19(4), 21–36.

Morse, J. M. (2001). Situating grounded theory. In R. S. Schreiber & P. Noerager Stern (Eds.), *Using grounded theory in nursing* (pp. 1–15). New York: Springer.

Morse, J. M. (2001). The cultural sensitivity of grounded theory [Editorial]. *Qualitative Health Research*, 11(6), 721–722.

Morse, J. M. (2007). Sampling in grounded theory research. In T. Bryant & K. Charmaz (Eds.), *Handbook of grounded theory* (pp. 229–244). London: Sage.

Morse J. M. & Bottorff, J. L. (1988). The emotional experience of breast expression. *Journal of Nurse-Midwifery*, 33(4), 165–170. Reprinted in 1992 in J. M. Morse (Ed.), *Qualitative health research* (pp. 319–332). Menlo Park, CA: Sage.

Morse, J. M. & Bottorff, J. L. (1989). Managing breastfeeding: The problem of leaking. *Journal of Nurse Midwifery*, 34(1), 15–20.

Morse, J. M. & Johnson, J. L. (Eds.). (1991). *The illness experience: Dimensions of suffering.* Newbury Park, CA: Sage. Available online at http://content.lib.utah.edu/u?/ir-main,2008 (accessed September 15, 2008).

Morse, J. M. & O'Brien, B. (1995). Preserving self: From victim, to patient, to disabled person. *Journal of Advanced Nursing*, 21, 886–896.

Wills, B. & Morse, J. M. (2008). Responses of Chinese elderly to the threat of severe acute respiratory syndrome (SARS) in a Canadian community. *Public Health Nursing.* 25(1), 57–68.

Wilson, S. & Morse, J. M. (1991). Living with a wife undergoing chemotherapy: Perceptions of the husband. *Image: Journal of Nursing Scholarship*, 23(2), 78–84. Reprinted in G. D. Wegner & R. J. Alexander (Eds.), *Readings in family nursing* (pp. 220–233). Philadelphia: J.B. Lippincott.

Wilson, S., Morse, J. M., & Penrod, J. (1998). Absolute involvement: The experience of mothers of ventilator-dependent children. *Health & Social Care*, 6(4), 224–233.

Phyllis Noerager Stern

Dr. Phyllis Stern graduated with her BS in nursing in 1970 from San Francisco State University. She received her MS in maternal-child nursing in 1971 and her DNS in family health in 1976, both from UCSF. This gives her the award for the longest collaboration with Barney Glaser of those who participated on the Bash panel.

Dr. Stern strayed from California. She has served as professor at Northwestern State University, Shreveport, Louisiana; as professor and director at Dalhousie University, Halifax, Canada; and is presently Professor Emerita at Indiana University. She has made a remarkable contribution to women's health, serving as the editor of *Health Care for Women International* for nineteen years and founding the International Council of Women's Health Issues.

In 2003, Dr. Stern was awarded Doctor of Laws honoris causa, Dalhousie University, Nova Scotia, Canada, for her contribution to the changing face of nursing in Eastern Canada. In 2008 she was named a "Living Legend" by the American Academy of Nursing.

Bibliography

Baker, C., & Stern, P. N. (1993). Finding meaning in chronic illness as a key to self care. *Canadian Journal of Nursing Research*, 25, 23–36.

Baker, C., Wuest, J., & Stern, P. N. (1992). Method slurring: The grounded theory/phenomenology example. *Journal of Advanced Nursing*, 17, 1355–1360. Republished in B. G. Glaser (Ed.), *Grounded theory 1984–1994*, vol. 1 (pp. 41–52). Mill Valley, CA: Sociology Press.

Dangdomyouth, P., Stern, P. N., Oumtanee, A. & Yunibhand, J. (2008). Tactful monitoring: How Thai caregivers manage their schizophrenic relatives at home. *Issues in Mental Health Nursing*, 29, 1, 37–50.

Dobrykowski, T. M. & Stern, P. N. (2003) Out of sync: A generation of first-time mothers over 30. *Health Care for Women International*, 24, 242–253.

Doyle, D. L. & Stern, P. N. (1992). Negotiating self care in rehabilitative nursing. *Rehabilitation Nursing*, 17, 319–321, 326.

Drauker, C. B. & Stern, P. N. (2000). Women's responses to sexual violence by male intimates. *Western Journal of Nursing Research*, 22, 385–496.

Keddy, B., Sims, S., & Stern, P. N. (1996). Grounded theory as feminist research methodology. *Journal of Advanced Nursing*, 23, 448–453.

Malloy, C. & Stern, P. N. (2000). Awakening as a change process among women at risk for HIV who engage in survival sex. *Qualitative Health Research*, 10, 581–594.

Mlay, R., Keddy, B., & Stern, P. N. (2004). Demands out of context: Tanzanian women combining exclusive breastfeeding while employed. *Health Care for Women International*, 25, 242–254.

Persley-Crotteau, S. & Stern, P. N. (1996). Creating a new life: Dimensions of temperance in perinatal cocaine crack users. *Qualitative Health Research*, 6, 152–162.

Pyles, S. H. & Stern, P. N. (1983). Discovery of nursing gestalt in critical care nursing: The importance of the gray gorilla syndrome. *Image*, 15, 51–57. Reprinted in B. G. Glaser (Ed.), *Grounded theory 1984–1994*, vol. 2 (pp. 447–465). Mill Valley, CA: Sociology Press.

Scheela, R. A. & Stern, P. N. (1994). Falling apart: A process essential to recovery in male incest offenders. *Archives of Psychiatric Nursing*, 8, 91–100.

Schreiber, R. & Stern, P. N. (Eds). (2001). *Using grounded theory in nursing.* New York: Springer. Translated into Korean in 2004.

Schreiber, R. & Stern, P. N. (Eds.). (2001). Using grounded theory to study women's health. *Health Care for Women International*, 22(1 & 2), Special issue.

Schreiber, R., Stern, P. N., & Wilson, C. (1998). The context for managing depression and its stigma among Black West Indian Canadian women. *Journal of Advanced Nursing*, 27, 510–517.

Stern, P. N. (1980). Grounded theory methodology: Its uses and processes. *Image*, 12, 20–23. Republished in S. R. Gortner (Ed.), *Nursing science methods* (pp. 79–88). San Francisco: University of California Press. Republished in B. G. Glaser (Ed.), *More grounded theory methodology* (pp. 116–126). Mill Valley, CA: Sociology Press.

Stern, P. N. (1982). Affiliating in stepfather families: Teachable strategies leading to integration. *Western Journal of Nursing Research*, 4, 75–89.

Stern, P. N. (1982). Conflicting family culture: An impediment to integration in stepfather families. *Journal of Psychosocial Nursing*, 20, 27–33. Reprinted in B. G. Glaser (Ed.), *Grounded theory 1984–1994*, vol. 2 (pp. 865–880). Mill Valley, CA: Sociology Press.

Stern, P. N. (1985). Using grounded theory in nursing research. In M. Leininger (Ed.), *Qualitative research methods in nursing* (pp. 149–160). New York: Grunne & Stratton.

Stern, P. N. (1986). *Women, health and culture.* New York: Hemisphere.

Stern, P. N. (Ed.). (1989). *Pregnancy & parenting.* New York: Hemisphere.

Stern, P. N. (1991). Are counting and coding a capella appropriate in qualitative research? In J. M. Morse (Ed.), *Qualitative nursing research: A contemporary dialogue* (pp. 135–148). Newbury Park, CA: Sage.

Stern, P. N. (1991). Women abuse and practice within an international context. In C. Sampselle (Ed.), *Violence against women* (pp. 143–152). New York: Hemisphere.

Stern, P. N. (Ed.). (1993). *Lesbian health care: What are the issues?* New York: Taylor & Francis.

Stern, P. N. (1994). Eroding grounded theory. In J. M. Morse (Ed.), *Critical issues in qualitative inquiry* (pp. 212–223). Newbury Park, CA: Sage. Spanish translation, University of Antioquia, 1994. Republished in B. G. Glaser (Ed.), *Grounded theory 1984–1994,* vol. 1 (pp. 53–64). Mill Valley, CA: Sociology Press.

Stern, P. N. (1996). Conceptualizing women's health: Discovering the dimensions. *Qualitative Health Research,* 6, 152–161.

Stern, P. N. (1996). Integrative discipline in stepfather families. In B. G. Glaser (Ed.), *Gerund grounded theory: The basic social process dissertation* (pp. 95–103). Mill Valley, CA: Sociology Press.

Stern, P. N. (2003). Founding and processes of the International Council on Women's Health Issues: Attentive partnering. The first 19 years. *Health Care for Women International,* 24, 271–279.

Stern, P. N., Allen, L. M., & Moxley, P. A. (1982). Qualitative research: The nurse as grounded theorist. *Health Care for Women International,* 4, 371–385.

Stern, P. N., Allen, L. M., & Moxley, P. A. (1982). The nurse as a grounded theorist: History, processes and uses. *The Review Journal of Philosophy and Social Science,* 7, 200–215. Reprinted in M. Belok & N. Haggerson (Eds.), *Naturalistic research paradigms* (pp. 200–215). Meerut, India: ANU.

Stern, P. N. & Covan, E. K. (2001). Early grounded theory: Its processes and products. In R. Schreiber & P. N. Stern (Eds.), *Using grounded theory in nursing* (pp. 17–34). New York: Springer.

Stern, P. N. & Kerry, J. (1996). Restructuring life after home loss by fire. *Image: The Journal of Nursing Scholarship,* 28, 9–14.

Stern, P. N. & Pyles, S. H. (1985). Using grounded theory methodology to study women's culturally based decisions about health. *Health Care for Women International,* 6, 1–24.

Stiffler, D., Sims, S. L., & Stern, P. N. (2007). Changing woman: Mothers and their adolescent daughters. *Health Care for Women International,* 28, 638–653.

Wuest, J., Ericson, P. K., & Stern, P. N. (1994). Becoming strangers: The changing family caregiving relationship in Alzheimer's disease. *Journal of Advanced Nursing,* 20, 437–443.

Wuest, J., Ericson, P., & Stern, P. (2001). Connected and disconnected support:

The impact on the caregiving process in Alzheimer's disease. *Health Care for Women International,* 22 (1/2), 115–130.

Wuest, J. & Stern, P. N. (1990). Impact of fluctuating relationships with the Canadian health care system on family management of otitis media with effusion. *Journal of Advanced Nursing,* 15, 556–563.

Wuest, J. & Stern, P. N. (1990). Childhood otitis media: The family's endless quest for relief. *Issues in Comprehensive Pediatric Nursing,* 13, 499–513.

DATE DUE

ILL# 5667 4839	FGM 9.23.09
ILL# 63400760	SYB 4-2-10
ILL# 84815740	AUM 1-3-12
ILL# 94459869	AUM 10.10.12
12/00/12 9750 7861	IAT
JAN 16 2014 ILL# 11827558	ANTCH
AUG 12 2015 IL 150933950	ANTCH

GAYLORD   PRINTED IN U.S.A.